THE NO EXCUSES DIET

"THE ANTI-DIET APPROACH TO CRANK UP YOUR ENERGY AND WEIGHT LOSS!

JONATHAN ROCHE

Award-Winning Fitness Expert, 12-time Ironman Triathlon Finisher and 17-time Boston Marathon Finisher"

ISBN: 1482603322
ISBN 13: 9781482603323

DEDICATION

To my beautiful wife Karen, your love and support is why I am the luckiest man in the world, to my wonderful boys Alexander and Benjamin, you make every day a gift, to my Dad, who struggled but gave everything he had to make our lives better and to my Mom, who made our short 12 years together truly magical!

ACKNOWLEDGMENTS

I would like to thank several people for their support, contributions, and guidance in writing this book.

I would like to thank my amazing wife Karen and my remarkable sons Alexander and Benjamin for letting me work so hard and long on this book.

I also want to thank my mother-in-law Mary Jo Alexander and father-in-law Jim Alexander for all their love and support.

In addition, I want to thank Carol Renaud for the love and support she showered on me since my Mom passed away in 1984.

To Eric Hajer, thanks for being a source of inspiration and knowledge and for convincing me to ditch my finance career in the late 90's.

To Chris Roche, Carolyn Compton and Don Roche, Jr., thanks for always believing in me since our childhood.

To the memory of Mary Ross, whose initial collaboration on this book was a starting point for me to gather and organize my ideas.

To David Perlick, Stephanie Louden, Tierney Smith, Franz Russell and Sean James, thanks for playing such important roles in how we empower and support our amazing members.

To Marla Ciley (The FlyLady) and Kelly Burns, thanks for being great friends and for giving my team and me the opportunity to serve all the FlyBabies.

To Tom Shook, Eric and Carrie Morrison, Mike and Betty Gay, Dennis Byrne, and Darius Baer, thanks for investing in my initial vision and for always being so supportive of our mission.

To Greg Farrington, Sven Anderson, Rory Hutchins, and Chris O'Brien, thanks for being true and remarkable friends and for all your support.

To Richard Del Maestro, my new close friend, professional speaking coach and audio director. Your brilliant insights, editing, writing and creative contributions took this book from merely representing my ideas to becoming a work that can transform millions of lives.

TABLE OF CONTENTS

EDITOR'S NOTE

My friend Darren Hardy first introduced me to Jonathan Roche as we were preparing for another interview I was recording for SUCCESS Magazine. As publisher of SUCCESS, Darren has deep relationships with more leading visionaries in the personal development field than one can possibly imagine. As we got ready for the interview with Jonathan I took note of Darren's particularly high level of enthusiasm for the upcoming conversation. He was animated, mentioned how Jonathan had encouraged his wife to run a half marathon, and told me just how much I'd like him because he was a truly great guy.

However, I didn't expect Darren's next comment. Just before the formal interview began he said to Jonathan, "Perhaps *you* can help Richard finally get in shape. I've tried and given up because he won't listen to me. Who knows, maybe he'll listen to you."

My struggles at the gym had already been well-documented and shared with millions of Darren Hardy's readers in his bestselling book *The Compound Effect* and in the magazine... under a supposedly false name. In fact, Darren used my real name in the story (and now you know the inside joke too). Well at the very least, you'd think that "public" humiliation would have finally broken through my resistance. Right? Nope.

In any case, Jonathan, the ever-compassionate fitness expert, leapt at the chance to help yet another physical fitness failure. And so when the interview concluded, our relationship began.

Jonathan was simply amazing right out of the gate. He was respectful and sensitive. He understood the all too common struggles I'd experienced sustaining a regular exercise program. Suddenly I found myself getting excited about a subject that I'd been avoiding and even dreading my entire life.

As a result of Darren Hardy's initial introduction I also had the privilege of being invited to work on this book. During the process of editing and recording the manuscript I've had the unusual opportunity to observe Jonathan as few have. I am inspired to share this experience with you because I want you to know something about Jonathan Roche you might not otherwise have a chance to learn.

While my credentials do not involve any expertise in the fields of fitness, nutrition or medicine, I have had a chance to watch Jonathan closely during the work we've done on this extraordinary book. I'd like to report my findings with the hope that you will learn to trust Jonathan just as much as I do.

As you will discover in these pages, Jonathan has done the research. His life's work has been to create a balanced and practical application of everything science has to offer about the strategic use of exercise and nutrition to achieve optimal health.

And he's been thorough, combing through the work of universities, behavioral scientists, medical doctors, exercise physiologists, nutritionists, sports psychologists and even life insurance statisticians to develop a truly holistic program that absolutely anyone can adopt.

However, what compelled me to write this is what I've observed about Jonathan while working intimately with him on this book. There *is a reason* Jonathan is able to help people who previously failed while dieting and exercising, and I believe my time with him has revealed that clearly.

If you were to ask me to describe his magnetic power in just one word, that word would have to be *character*. Jonathan is among the most compassionate, sincere and loving people I've met. Moreover, in the fifty-plus hours we spent together recording his audiobook, Jonathan never lost sight of why he was working so hard on his message. His selfless motivation was obvious from the moment we began to the moment we had completed our time together. It was extraordinary to behold.

Not only has he been a joy to record, to write with, to edit with, and to coach, he has been a joy to spend time with in general. If you could share the privilege of watching Jonathan greet a stranger at Starbucks or speak with someone across the counter at a restaurant, perhaps you'd understand why I wanted to write this note. Watching Jonathan interact with people he's never met before is a lesson in kindness and empathy that all of us could use.

I'm hoping he'll let me print this in spite of his epic humility, because if you'll trust my words, and just take a chance of surrendering your health and diet goals to Jonathan's guidance, you will join the growing thousands who would have to agree that Jonathan is destined to be deemed America's Fitness Coach.

Sure, I believe he's got the weight-loss answers, and I think you'll have to concur if you study this book with all sincerity. But what truly sets him apart is his deepest heartfelt desire to help you, me and literally everyone he meets.

The man is utterly non-judgmental. When he looks at someone who is obese, has terrible self-esteem, and perhaps even a bit of self-loathing, all Jonathan seems capable of seeing is a beautiful person and an opportunity to be of help. His x-ray vision seems to go straight to the heart. Again, I only wish you could have joined us for coffee. If you had, you'd be nodding your head in agreement right now.

My advice, after working with him intimately for so many hours is this: trust Jonathan Roche. Trust his advice, trust his system, and most of all trust his motivation. I would sign up to put my name and reputation on the line for him in a heartbeat, anywhere and anytime. Once you meet him in person, through his online videos, through the audio and print version of this book, on his radio show and on TV, I know you'll have to agree with me wholeheartedly that he's utterly worth your trust as well.

My hope is that these words will help you start this book with an open mind and heart, and thus have a greater chance of following Jonathan's lead. In the short time I've implemented his advice I've gotten into the best shape ever. As of this writing I've completed fifty-five consecutive days of working out, and it's changing my life. My family and friends can see the difference and my energy, stamina and health has skyrocketed. Thanks Jonathan.

So dear reader congratulations on finding the fitness opportunity of a lifetime. Now I'd like to introduce you to your new best friend. I call him America's Fitness Coach, Jonathan Roche.

Richard Del Maestro

INTRODUCTION

Are You Surviving, Living, or Thriving?

Surviving: You have no energy, you have to drink coffee or soda all day, you never or rarely exercise, and you generally feel terrible. You are just trying to make it through your day and are usually dragging. This is zero fun and no way to live!

Living: You feel OK—not good and not bad. You don't have tons of energy, but you can generally make it through the day with coffee in the morning and maybe an occasional soda in the afternoon. You exercise inconsistently but generally fit in two to four workouts per week. This is not a bad place to be, but the opportunity to have more energy and feel truly great is only a few key moves away.

Thriving: You are on fire and have limitless energy! You can play with your kids for hours or go for a long walk or hike with a friend without even thinking about it. You are nailing five or six workouts per week. You have a ton of self-confidence, are truly healthy, and jump out of bed each morning ready to tackle the day. This is a magical place to be, as you feel amazing and your kids and family are drawing positive energy from you being a healthy role model. Life is great!

Are you surviving, living, or thriving?

If you are surviving, then it's time to start living!

If you are living, then it is time to start thriving!

And once you start thriving, believe me, you will never turn back!

Life it too short to just survive or live. Now is your time to thrive so lets get started!

Why I'm Excited to Lead You

I was 224 pounds, wearing size thirty-eight pants, working long hours, and generally dragging along back in 1995 when my dad (who was obese and struggled with his weight and health) died suddenly of cardiac arrest. That was my wake-up call. I realized that my family needed me, and taking care of my health was too important to avoid—and the same is true for you!

My father was a great guy, and I would have loved for my two sons (Alexander and Benjamin) to have met and been influenced by him. But my dad only met one out of his nine grandchildren because he didn't have the tools to lose weight and get healthy. His heart was in the right place, and he tried many different diets and programs to lose weight. But he couldn't keep the weight off because the diets and programs were not sustainable, and inevitably he would go back to his old habits. This book is the program my dad needed and deserved, and that's why I am so excited to share it with you!

If Not Now, When?

Consider what your New Year's resolutions were for this year—and whether or not you are in the process of chasing them down. Have you reached your goals? If you are like most people the answer is no.

Now I have a challenge for you: I want you to take a few minutes right now (not later today, not tomorrow but right now) to consider what you have been thinking about doing (losing fifty pounds, walking your first 5K, running your first marathon, etc.) and commit to starting on that journey right now!

We all have things we talk about doing, but most of us keep putting them off and never make them happen. We let the days become months, then years, and ultimately those fitness and weight-loss goals remain unattained. But the key question is this: If not now, when?

Honestly, think about it for a minute.

We don't live forever, and none of us is getting any younger. The idea that life will slow down and free us to take action is only a dream. I'm not saying this to drag you down but to cut to the chase. I want you to realize that every day you let pass by not chasing down your dreams and goals is another day lost. Once a day passes, you can't get it back. So let me ask you this again: If not now, when?

Is Today the Day?

Is today the day when everything changes? Is today the day when you finally say enough is enough?

Is today the day you realize that you're worth it and that you deserve to have unlimited energy and feel like a million bucks? Is today the day that you realize the extra weight you have carried around for years (maybe even decades) has robbed you of becoming who you deserve to be?

As I mentioned earlier, we don't live forever (the average US life expectancy is seventy-eight years, so you can do the math). I don't say that to scare you but to add some realistic immediacy to the need to make your health a top priority. Life is too short to waste time having low energy and feeling bad!

I invite you to take a few minutes to think about the above questions and then to respond with a solid "yes" and follow my lead. You'll shock yourself with what you accomplish and who you become! Make today *the* day!

15 Secrets to Better Health

This book is mostly focused on winning the mental game as far as getting fit and losing weight. Use these 15 habits as your "What do I actually do?" Guide while you work your way through the book. With the one-two combination of Strong Mental Muscles and these 15 habits you will be unstoppable!

OK, it's time to print out the 15 Secrets to Better Health (you can get the list by going to www.NoExcuses Workouts.com/Book). Then review them and focus on doing the easiest five for you right away for one week. Then add one more from the list each week. I suggest you post this list on your fridge so that you see it every day.

15 Secrets to Better Health

Attitude and Focus

1) **Concentrate on your health as opposed to losing weight.** If you have kids, concentrate on your kids and how your losing weight will help improve the energy you bring to your relationship with them.
2) **Hold yourself accountable, and don't make excuses.** We're all extremely busy, but you can fit movement into your schedule. You deserve to take some personal time each day to invest in yourself and your health.
3) **When you exercise, be proud of yourself.** Know how much it positively affects your energy and health.
4) **Stay positive.** Life's too short to beat yourself up over weight you've gained or workouts you've missed. Staying positive helps all areas of your life.
5) **Have fun.** If your workouts aren't fun, you aren't going to keep doing them. So, if you dread going to a gym, don't go. Instead, go for a walk, play with your kids in the yard, etc. If you can turn the dreaded "exercise" word into a fun activity,

then your chances of being successful increase dramatically.

6) **Throw the rearview mirror out the window.** Concentrate on today and tomorrow. You can't change the past, and beating yourself up is only going to drag you in the wrong direction. Today is a new day!

Exercise and Movement

7) **Do Interval Workouts three days per week.** Intervals help you burn 30 percent more calories per workout and can help leave your metabolism elevated for up to twelve hours after each workout. You can access a free sample workout by going to: http://www.NoExcusesWorkouts.com/Book
8) **Do the six-minute No Excuses workout three days per week.** You can do this quick and highly effective strength-training workout right in your living room; no equipment is required. You can access the free sample workout by going to: http://www.NoExcusesWorkouts.com/Book
9) **Perform Random Acts of Fitness.** Take the stairs at work, park in the farthest spot in the parking lot, play with your kids instead of sitting on the sidelines, walk in place while brushing your teeth, etc. Be creative and you can turn activities you already do into opportunities to improve your health.

Nutrition

10) **Always eat breakfast, and never skip meals.** Have breakfast within one hour of waking up to kick-start your metabolism. Skipping meals causes your metabolism to slow down. It sends the signal to

your body to store your next meal as fat in order to avoid starving.

11) **Drink sixty-four ounces of water per day** plus one additional ounce per minute of workout time. You should be going to the bathroom at least once every hour to hour and a half.
12) **Eat something every two to three hours.** Eat healthy snacks midmorning and midafternoon to help keep your metabolism buzzing and avoid overeating at lunch or dinner.
13) **Control your portions.** Avoid seconds and eat until you're no longer hungry versus until you are full.
14) **Only have dessert once per week.** This could save you 400 calories per day on your six non-dessert days and that adds up to 2,400 calories per week. Since you have to burn 3,500 more calories than you consume to lose one pound, this one new habit alone could lead to losing an additional pound every two weeks, or 36 pounds in one year!
15) **Limit yourself to one soda per day (ideally zero per day).** The excess sugar isn't good for your health and soda consumption will cause major ups and downs in your level of energy throughout the day.

CHAPTER 1: THE FREEDOM OF A FRESH START

DON'T LOSE HOPE

If you look up the word "hope" in *Webster's Dictionary* you will find this definition: "The feeling that what is wanted can be had or that events will turn out for the best."

Take a moment right now to consider whether you feel like you've lost hope when it comes to reaching your goal weight and goal fitness level.

Maybe you've had challenging experiences in the past with trying to get fit and lose weight (crazy diets, insane exercise plans, being fooled into thinking taking a pill will work, etc.). These experiences become part of your history, part of your fitness-and-weight-loss story. In fact, these negative experiences often fuel your negative voice, which can become overwhelming and begin to dictate the path you are taking on your journey. Your negative voice begins to decide for you if you can accomplish your next goal. It begins to take the power away from the actual driver of the car: *you*.

If your negative voice is lecturing you right now, saying, "You aren't going to pull this off," then take comfort in the fact that you've never tried to lose weight and get fit with the approach you'll learn in this book. You can create a new and better path. *You* are the driver.

If you've lost hope, then I have some great news. We're going to work on getting rid of that negative voice. We're going to learn to focus on the present, on the things we can do in the now to change where we're going in our future. Follow my lead in this book, and you'll grab control of the wheel. Before long you'll be driving down the road to a new and better life!

Then, not only will you have hope but you will also eventually accomplish your fitness and weight-loss goals. This is not a dream—it's the truth.

You deserve to have tons of energy and to feel amazing, so have hope and get ready to shock yourself with who you become. Now is your time!

YOUR WEIGHT ISN'T WHO YOU ARE

The actions you've taken in the past—good or bad (exercise, eating habits, etc.)—are what have led to your current weight. Therefore, your weight today is a culmination of decisions that are now water under the bridge. You can't do anything to change these decisions since they're in the past. What you can do is make yourself and your health a top priority, starting right now, so that your future weight (next week, the end of this year, etc.) is different.

Here's the key question: Are you ready to make you and your health a top priority?

The day you answer this with a screaming "yes!" is the day that your life will change forever!

If this question scares you "Are you ready to make you and your health a top priority?", that's good. Consider this: When was the last time you did something great without being scared?

Change can be challenging but in this case it is a sign of your potential for personal growth!

YOUR PAST IS NOT YOUR FUTURE

As you focus on getting fit and losing weight, your negative voice will try to convince you that "this attempt" isn't going to work. It'll try to come up with evidence of past failures and frustrations that will make you question whether you can succeed this time. I want you to remember this:

Your past is not your future!

Just because you've made other attempts to get fit and lose weight that didn't work out (which only means you're human) doesn't mean that this attempt can't be different.

Too many people label themselves based on their past, particularly when it comes to weight loss, and you deserve better. There's nothing you can do about decisions you've already made, so hammering yourself about weight you've gained, workouts you've missed, or food you ate only takes you in the wrong direction. In fact, when you spend time (any time) thinking about yesterday's missteps, you're using energy that you could be putting into winning today.

I have an important request. Don't let yesterday's missteps rob you of today's and tomorrow's victories! Give yourself permission right now to forget your past experiences with fitness and weight loss.

Once you do that, you free yourself to put 100 percent of your energy into winning today by focusing on things you can do *starting immediately* to improve your health. And it's simple: You can drink water, eat every two to three hours, park far from the door at the grocery store, fit in your workout and be grateful for the gift of being able to walk. And as we will talk about later, gratitude goes a long way toward building healthy habits!

In order to get a realistic picture of what you've been focusing on each day, please complete the following exercise. Give percentages of the amount of time during an average day that you spend focusing on each of these:

The Past: looking back at yesterday (or being lectured by your negative voice about missed workouts, bad nutritional choices, weight you have put back on, etc.)

The Present: today (how much water have I had, when am I working out, etc.)

The Future: looking forward (How am I going to lose thirty pounds by the end of the year? What if I can't stay consistent for the entire month?)

Honestly rate each of these, and then spend two minutes looking at your answers and thinking about them.

What would happen to your fitness and weight-loss results if you put 100 percent of your energy into today? What would this do for your mental peace of mind? What would this do as far as reducing your stress?

When (not if) you put 100 percent of your energy into making today amazing and nailing your healthy habits, amazing things will happen, and your rocket will leave the pad!

Embrace the fact that today is a new day and that you can't do anything to change yesterday - but that you can put all your effort into winning today.

THROW YOUR REARVIEW MIRROR OUT THE WINDOW

I have another challenge for you that'll help you get rid of your negative voice. Spend the next twenty-four hours without saying anything negative about yourself or anyone else. Yes, I'm serious. Honestly try this. What you'll learn is just how much your negative voice is talking you down.

As we discussed earlier, the majority of the noise is about your past. I invite you to throw your rearview mirror out the window! Beating yourself up only drags you in the wrong direction. There's nothing you can do about any of that, so concentrate on today. Focus on looking forward and not on what's behind you.

HIT THE RESTART BUTTON

The idea of a restart button can be a powerful one. Haven't we all had days when we'd like to just start over again? What if we could do that for bigger things, like health and weight loss?

OK, so you had grand New Year's resolutions that have already faded. Maybe you wanted to reach a certain weight or be able to accomplish some type of fitness activity by a certain date, but it just didn't happen.

You now have two options:

Listen to your negative voice as it lectures you about how you failed—blah, blah, blah...

or

Say, "OK, I bailed on my healthy habits, but today is a new day and I'm going to hit the restart button."

The second option is what you and your family deserve. Being lectured all day by your negative voice is zero fun, and it holds you back and keeps you from continuing your pursuit of your goals. Like I said, throw away that rearview mirror! Life is too short, so hit your restart button today.

MAKE TODAY JANUARY 1

Many people put a big emphasis on starting a new fitness and weight-loss plan on January 1. While it's always great to have goals for specific time lines, this particular one has become too powerful and makes people discouraged when they're not successful. It also can lead to thinking that if you didn't stick to your plan during the first weeks of the New Year, you should just give up.

Research shows that 80 percent of people bail on their New Year's resolutions by the end of week two, and 98 percent bail by the end of week four! Why do we think that we "blew it" because on one particular day we made grand plans for how much weight we would lose this year? Why wait until January 1 to start doing amazing things with your energy and health?

If you started the year with solid intentions and never got going or have fallen off, then today is a great day to start. Any day can be the start of something amazing, so make today your January 1. Forget about however many weeks have passed this year—that's now water under the bridge.

Remember, focusing on yesterday is something you can't change and is only going to drag you in the wrong direction. Jump in and make today your January 1. Then get excited to crush it over the remaining weeks of the year!

TAKE YOUR SECOND CHANCE

My brother, Chris, has endured a great deal throughout his life. He was diagnosed with a rare form of nose cancer at the young age of thirty-five, and he thought it was all over. He is a very positive guy, but it wasn't looking good, as the cancer grew from his nose up almost to his brain. After fighting through thirty surgeries over four years, and having his nose and part of his face removed, he came out the other side. He is embracing his second chance!

When you almost die, it changes everything—it wakes you up. You don't need to fight off a deadly disease to embrace the concept of a second chance.

Maybe you're disappointed with the weight you've gained over the years, and you know in your heart that you're better than that. The sad but important truth is that we aren't going to live forever.

Stop waiting for the perfect time to take action (you'll be waiting for the rest of your life) and instead take your second chance starting right now!

If you have a lot of weight to lose or are out of shape, view today as your "second chance." You have an open day and future to build the life of your dreams and to write a new story—so grab it and take advantage of it. Your health is truly a gift, so take your second chance!

TURN FEAR INTO YOUR SECRET WEAPON

Fear of failure robs many people of the fitness and weight-loss success they deserve. Their negative voices convince them that it's less risky to keep doing what they're doing rather than risk the humiliation of not being successful in their efforts to lose weight and get fit.

But the sad thing is that this is a complete lie!

First, the only true failure is staying down. More than likely you'll experience setbacks along the way (you're human), but as long as you keep getting back up, you're learning. With enough persistence and the right tools (especially the mental ones you'll learn in this book), success will be yours.

Second, the people who would judge you if you were to "fail" are not people you want to be friends with anyway. Why waste your time worrying about being judged? Your fans (your friends and family) who truly care about you don't judge you.

Third, most of our fears never come true anyway. We spend all this time worrying about whether something is going to happen or not, and 90 percent of the time, none of it materializes.

Fourth, you've never attempted to get fit and lose weight by wrestling control of the podium from your negative voice and combining that with quick and powerful workouts and simple daily habits! So although your negative voice will feed you lines like "Haven't you tried this before and quit?" the truthful answer is no. You haven't tried "this" before because "this" is completely different and sustainable.

It's time to turn fear into your secret weapon!

Warning: This is going to get bumpy for a few minutes, so please tell your negative voice to take a hike so that you can work through this.

The word "potential" is defined in *Webster's Dictionary* as "Existing in possibility: Capable of development into actuality." Here's something very exciting: we're all only using a small portion of our true potential!

I'm not saying this to freak you out or give your negative voice more material to lecture you about. I'm saying this because it's a good thing that should get you excited about the future. I suggest from this moment forward that you shift from fearing failure to fearing not reaching your potential.

Just reading this should make you a bit uncomfortable because most people want nothing to do with talking about reaching their potential. But what if instead of running from the concept of reaching your potential, you ran toward it? What if each day you thought about how you could take actions that led you closer and closer to your true potential?

Your negative voice will try to convince you that it can't be this simple and that your time is better spent dwelling on the past. But at this point you know that's the road to nowhere.

Here's the fun part: the less of your potential you've reached so far, the more fired up you should be about your future because of the tremendous progress you are going to make!

There is no greater regret later in life than not having lived up to your potential. The great thing is that you're not ninety years old sitting on the porch telling your spouse about all your regrets. You now have the time to change the outcome, and this should get you excited to take action.

If you'll give yourself the gift of converting your fear of failure into a fear of not living up to your potential, then you'll have discovered a secret weapon in your pursuit of becoming who you deserve to be!

CHAPTER 2: QUICK FIXES DON'T WORK

THERE IS NO EFFECTIVE QUICK FIX

"There are no shortcuts to any place worth going."
—Beverly Sills

This is *not* a quick-fix program. My approach to healthy and sustained weight loss is to avoid quick fixes, take baby steps, and build true and lasting changes in your behavior and routines. Losing weight and getting fit require hard work and sweat. Don't let that intimidate you—it's just the truth.

If you think you can pop a weight-loss pill and sit on the couch to lose weight and keep it off, you're in for a huge disappointment. Please ditch the dream of using a quick fix to lose weight and get fit. You only set yourself up for failure and a letdown, and you deserve better than that.

Even if you could safely pop a pill and lose weight while sitting on the couch, it would still be too risky to be inactive from a health standpoint. In fact, being inactive makes you vulnerable to the same health risks as smokers. According to the American Heart Association, "The relative risk of coronary heart disease associated with physical inactivity is comparable to high cholesterol, high blood pressure, or cigarette smoking."

What does this say about the person who's skinny through being "genetically lucky" and doesn't seem to need exercise? It says that her or his health is at risk (and the scary thing is, most people who fall into this category have no idea). I normally stay away from scary medical information because it isn't in line with the positive vibe we've created with our No Excuses team. But this information is extremely important.

Yes, fitting into your skinny jeans and losing weight are fun experiences. But the real victory (besides having tons of energy and feeling great) is being healthy and having a long and enjoyable life. That's what we all deserve, and we can earn it every day by staying active and making smart food choices.

95% OF DIETS FAIL

The high failure rate of diets is exactly why the No Excuses Diet is not a "diet." You've probably tried many diets but haven't been able to stick with them and you probably beat yourself up about not being able to follow through on those diets every time. Well, it's time to let all of that go!

Why do most diets fail? You actually set yourself up for failure when you go on a traditional diet or as I like to say, an excuse-based diet. Why? Because traditional diets are difficult to maintain and deprive your body of needed nutrients and/or favorite foods, which eventually drives you crazy leading to a bunch of excuses. And the excuses ultimately cause you to break the diet and fail. In addition, constantly being hungry can make you irritable, which is challenging for you and your family (especially your kids). Ever hear this one: I am really sorry but you are going to need to be more understanding. I am on a diet!

So, what can you do to stop making excuses, lose weight and keep it off?

We'll focus on these tips in greater detail later in the book, but the two major components of healthy weight loss include good and easily sustained nutrition (including the smart timing of when you take in nutrients) and healthy and effective exercise, focused on quality not quantity. Refer to the Fifteen Secrets to Better Health for the specific habits to build.

CALORIES IN CALORIES OUT VERSUS DIET PILLS

I cringe every time I see a diet-pill or quick-fix commercial geared towards Americans' obsession with quick weight loss. Americans spend $14 *billion* per year on diet pills! That's an average of forty-five dollars per American per year! Please don't waste your money on diet pills! There's a healthier and safer way to accomplish your weight-loss goals. Ninety-nine percent of diet pills aren't regulated by the FDA, which means you don't really know if they're safe or if the claims being made are accurate.

When it comes to weight loss and weight maintenance, it all comes down to calories burned versus calories consumed. To effectively lose weight and keep it off, you need to burn more calories than you consume.

- To lose one pound, you need to burn 3,500 more calories than you consume.
- To lose one pound per week (or fifty-two pounds in a year), you need to burn 500 more calories than you consume each day.

I want you to really think about how much healthier it is to approach weight loss from the standpoint of cranking up your metabolism through exercise—and most importantly Interval Workouts—and balancing that with smart nutrition. You don't need to waste your money on diet pills.

I'm not an expert on diet pills, nor am I a nutritionist, but I personally don't suggest that anyone take diet pills due to the lack of FDA regulation. Your health and safety are too important to risk.

If you question this advice, please Google "ephedra deaths" or "phen-fen deaths" to read about the deaths and health issues these diet pills caused. Instead of looking for a pill to do the job, focus on keeping active and watching your portion sizes. Being active has so many benefits that are worth every minute of time invested—more energy, improved self-esteem, being an example of health to your kids, and of course, a quicker metabolism to help you drop those pounds.

CLOSE THE GAP

There's a gap between where you are right now and where you want and deserve to be. And focusing on closing this gap is where all the magic happens!

Yes, you'll see movement in the scale. Yes, you'll get fitter. And yes, you will improve your health. But the true victory is that time spent closing the gap helps you realize that this whole thing is really about enjoying the journey and not about a destination.

"Look at what you can become in pursuit of
what you want."
—Jim Rohn

Most people are 100 percent focused on the outcome when they set a goal and take action to turn it into an accomplishment. And we will discuss how to set and achieve your goals later on in the book. But the hidden benefit is who you become while pursuing the goal.

ARE YOU GOING ON VACATION OR MOVING?

When you go on vacation, you're in a major hurry to get there the first day. You have no time to waste because your vacation days are limited. You go on vacation knowing that it will end and you must leave.

Moving is different! Yes, you want to get to where you're moving, but you aren't in the same type of rush as when you're leaving for vacation. When it comes to your fitness and weight-loss journey, are you going on vacation or moving? Is this an enlightening question? Yes. So ask yourself now: Why are you stressing so much about the speed with which you get to your destination if you're honestly moving there and will be there for the rest of your life?

Your negative voice will try to tell you that you should be bummed out if you "only" lost a pound last week. But when you're planning on staying at your goal weight (moving there) for the rest of your life, you should be fired up if you're losing one pound per week.

Why do you let your negative voice convince you that losing one pound per week is not enough? How about half a pound per week? Yes, I'm pushing you to shoot for losing one to three pounds per week, but if you drop one pound per week you'll lose fifty-two pounds in one year! That is rock-star status! Even half a pound per week would put you at an amazing twenty-six pounds lost in just one year.

BABY STEPS VERSUS CLIMBING MOUNT EVEREST

We live in an instant-gratification society—we want to lose 4 to 5 pounds per week. Losing 1 or 2 pounds per week makes it seem like it'll take you forever to lose the 25, 50, 100, or 150 pounds that you want to lose. Remember, however, that you did not get out of shape over the course of a few weeks or even months. More than likely you have been gaining weight gradually over a long period of time.

At any given time, you're only one decision away from starting to improve your health. So take your first step today by committing to moving and improving your health, one baby step at a time. By taking baby steps, you won't hurt yourself or get discouraged because you feel beat up.

Baby steps like drinking enough water, not skipping meals, and being grateful will add up. These actions positively affect your health. I want you to concentrate on taking positive baby steps each day versus concentrating on having to lose X amount of weight.

If you concentrate on having to lose fifty pounds (or whatever you want to lose), it's like standing at the bottom of Mount Everest and psyching yourself out with the magnitude of having to climb to the top. You deserve to feel amazing, so focus on taking baby steps each day, and then get ready to be shocked by your results.

DON'T SPRINT AT THE BEGINNING

If you're just starting your fitness routine, the worst thing you can do is sprint right out of the gate. If you do too much too soon, then you can burn out and potentially get injured. The key is to start slowly and take a long-term approach. You don't need to be a rock star this week or next; you just need to take baby steps and make healthy choices each day.

Also, if you're just starting out, you should be OK with the fact that you're going to feel exhausted for a few weeks and have to fight the negative self-talk in order to keep focused and moving forward.

Let me explain with an example from my own life. During a ten-mile Boston Marathon training run, I took a beating. Instead of getting discouraged and letting my negative voice drag me down ("How could you be this out of shape so close to the marathon?" "You're running so slowly!"), I just put one foot in front of the other and kept moving. The next weekend I did a twelve-mile run and didn't feel much better than the prior weekend. But again, I took it slow, kept moving, and finished. I didn't quit! This was challenging for me, but I was able to convince myself to ignore my negative voice and focus on the "big picture."

The following Saturday I did a fourteen-mile run and felt great! By taking a long-term approach over those few challenging weeks, I didn't get discouraged. My body was able to adapt, and I was able to gain confidence that I'd have a great day in the upcoming marathon. And this approach can apply to you no matter what level you are at!

If you're new to fitness, take a long-term approach, and remember that you don't need to sprint out of the gate. You just need to take it one baby step, one workout, and one healthy decision at a time, and before you know it, you'll be feeling great.

Remember, your journey to a healthier and more energized place is like a marathon: don't sprint out of the gate, stay consistent with your workouts and you will definitely reach your finish line.

EMBRACE REASONS TO WIN

So many people have failed at attempting to lose weight and get fit in the past that they approach each new attempt as though they're expecting it to not work.

Is that you?

My approach to helping you lose weight and get fit is different from anything you've tried before; it is based on proven research, smart choices and smart timing!

Let's make this your last attempt to get fit and lose weight because *you are going to pull it off* and make true lifestyle changes!

Of course, you can't sit on the couch eating chips and take a pill to lose weight. And yes, sweating is part of working out. So put aside the idea of losing four or five pounds per week. And follow my lead, lose one to two pounds per week (maybe three) and, most importantly, *keep it off forever.*

I want you to focus 100 percent of your energy on embracing reasons why this time you *are* going to lose weight, get fit, and keep it off for good. Forget about looking for reasons to fail (I missed a workout, I ate a whole pint of Ben & Jerry's, etc.). You deserve to feel good about yourself now! This is where the transformation begins!

EMBRACE THE CHALLENGE OF LOSING WEIGHT

Losing weight isn't easy. If it were, then 70 percent of the US would not be overweight. The hard facts are that you have to exercise regularly and make healthy food choices to lose a realistic and sustainable one to three pounds per week. Skipping dessert, taking the stairs, parking far from the door, and not having seconds of your favorite dinner are all challenging decisions. Fitting your workout into your busy schedule or making yourself do something active when you're tired is a challenging decision.

Instead of becoming intimidated by the challenges, I say embrace them and make them work for you! In the end, the victory of hitting your goal weight, finishing your first 5K, fitting into your skinny jeans, or most importantly having unlimited energy and being the example of health to your children is that much sweeter because the journey was challenging.

Also, since this program is about making smart nutritional choices and about taking a healthy approach to exercise that doesn't feel like a part-time job you will maximize your chances of success, you won't be overwhelmed and this will actually fit into your life. There's nothing fancy involved, just a highly effective, healthy, and sustainable approach to losing weight and getting in great shape!

So when your negative voice keeps complaining about how tough it is to lose weight, say to yourself the following:

"Yes, it is hard and that is OK. Look at other great things have I accomplished in life that were challenging when I started!"

Invest your energy in yourself - You're worth it! So embrace the struggle, avoid making excuses, and turn your fitness and weight-loss goals into victories!

CHAPTER 3: NOW IS YOUR TIME

YOU AREN'T GOING TO LIVE FOREVER

Did you ever notice how 90 percent of people complete their taxes in the last week prior to the April 15 deadline? They keep putting them off until they realize that they're out of time, so they finally take action.

Unfortunately, many people approach losing weight and getting healthy the same way. They continuously put it off until they have a health scare or realize later in life that they were robbed of decades of true happiness due to their weight—just as they're running out of time.

The average US life expectancy is 78 years. Unfortunately if you're overweight (one to thirty pounds) that number drops to 74.5, and if you're obese (thirty-plus pounds overweight), the number drops to 71 years. If you question the second two facts, then consider this: When's the last time you saw an obese seventy- or eighty-year-old?

Many people avoid the tough fact that we don't live forever. They spend their lives not making their health a priority and taking an "I'll lose the weight at some point" attitude. By the time they realize later in life that they blew it, it's too late. Life has passed them by, and they missed out on far too much by being out of shape and overweight or obese. You deserve better than that!

One example of people dreading the passage of time is that many adults don't enjoy their birthdays. How often have we heard (or felt!), "I can't believe I'm thirty, forty, or fifty," "Where did these gray hairs come from," or "Where did the last year, five years, or ten years go"? Birthdays, especially milestone birthdays (thirty, forty, fifty, etc.) often turn into a time to reflect on what we've done with our lives and where we are as far as meeting our life goals. If you're fit and feel amazing, birthdays turn into celebrations rather than painful evaluations!

Listen, I've been in the best shape of my life on each of my birthdays since 1996 when I dropped 40 pounds.

How do you want to celebrate your next birthday? Trust me, I know what it feels like to be out of shape and not feel good about yourself. Do you know what I mean? Life's too short to have low energy, to lack self-esteem, to be unhealthy, and to feel exhausted all the time. You can do this! Now is your time to make your health a top priority and to start feeling like a million bucks! Commit to making your next birthday (and all the ones that follow) a celebration. Join forces with me and lets make it happen!

THERE IS NO REPEAT BUTTON

Although we do get a restart button when it comes to deciding to start today, life doesn't come with a repeat button when it comes to time. Once a day, a week, a month, or a year passes, it's gone and can't be retrieved. Yet many people act as if they have a bank of unlimited days to pull from as far as chasing down their fitness and weight-loss goals. They tell themselves they'll get fit and lose weight when the timing is right. There are so many excuses: "I'll start Monday." "I'll get back on the workouts when the kids are back in school." "I have too much going on right now." Sound familiar?

The bottom line is that dreaming about a "right time" will leave you waiting forever. Our lives are nuts today, and they're going to be nuts tomorrow; so let go of the right-time dream and hit the gas *today*.

Life is flying by like sand slipping through your fingers. Stop hitting the "put it off" button and hit the "now is my time" button. Fitness and weight-loss results are the reward of action! I am telling it to you straight, stay with me now!

NO REGRETS NOW OR LATER

In the later years of life, it's a common theme that we don't regret what we did as much as we regret what we didn't do. Imagine yourself later in life having the opportunity to talk to yourself right now. What would you say?

Now is the time to set yourself up for having no regrets later in life. Every day that passes without your making your health and fitness a top priority is another day gone. The days become weeks become months become years become regrets.

Don't look back later in life and kick yourself, saying, "How many years was I robbed of and how many great experiences did I miss by not taking control of my health and weight?" You're better than that, and you deserve better. Now is the time to take action!

WHEN WAS THE LAST TIME YOU FELT AMAZING?

Honestly, really think about this question for a minute. Was the last time you felt amazing at your wedding? Was it before you had your first child? How long ago was it? Think back to how great you felt and how much energy you had.

How much would it impact your life to have limitless energy and limitless enthusiasm about: your kids, your spouse and your activities? This is how I feel every day and so do thousands of others we have helped with this very system. It's completely realistic for you to get back to that place. Yes, your life is more complex right now since you may have kids, own a home, or whatever, but I can guide you back to that amazing place of feeling like a million bucks if you follow my lead and take action.

Don't put off revealing the high-energy and healthy version of yourself that lies within. Most people never reach their potential and instead just accept going with the flow. As I mentioned previously, they keep putting off their dreams and goals until one day later in life they start asking themselves hard questions like "What could I have done or who could I have become if I'd just gone for it?"

Don't let that be you. Every one of us has unique greatness in us that is ready to be unlocked. Visualize having unlimited energy and the confidence and health to chase down your dreams, and then get after it!

BE COMMITTED, NOT JUST INTERESTED

I love the following quote and suggest you read it several times:

"There's a difference between interest and commitment. When you're interested in doing something, you do it only when it's convenient. When you're committed to something, you accept no excuses, only results."
— Author Unknown

When you're committed, you don't let your negative voice convince you that you don't have time to exercise when you spend time watching TV and online (for non-work purposes) each day. When you're committed, you follow my suggestions like setting yourself up for success each night by preparing a water bottle, workout clothes, and healthy snacks for the next day, even though you're tired and just want to relax on the couch with a glass of wine. When you're committed, you're confident that you will achieve your weight-loss goals because you take 100 percent ownership of your weight and your results.

You get the point. Make a true commitment today, and then make this year the launching pad for the new you. You're worth it!

DESTINED FOR GREATNESS

I read the words "Destined for Greatness" on a burp cloth that my wife, Karen, pulled out for our youngest son one morning when he was a baby. I loved seeing it. It made me think about the fact that when we're young, we're told that we can do anything we set our minds to: we're given the impression that we are "destined for greatness." While this is actually true, we do all have the potential to achieve greatness, somewhere along the way we often pull back on shooting for the moon and instead just go with the flow.

What big dreams do you have asleep inside of you? Have you dreamed of finishing a 5K, a 10K or even a marathon? Have you dreamed of having unlimited energy or being a healthy role model to your kids? Every one of us has had big dreams at some point. Every one of us has the strength inside to accomplish anything we set our minds to. You were destined for greatness when you were born, and I know today is the day to begin dreaming big again and then making those dreams happen. Yes you can!

CHAPTER 4: SET AND CHASE DOWN SCARY GOALS

WHY NOT YOU?

I was listening to one of my motivational CDs on the way home from the office, and the late Jim Rohn (whom I am a big fan of and have already quoted many times in this book) was talking about the concept of "why not you?"

This inspired me to talk to you about the fact that most of us look at successful people without realizing that we to have the opportunity to define our lives and our health just as they have. Yes, we all have various challenges we've dealt with in the past or are currently dealing with. But the reality is that we all have an opportunity right now to take control of our health and improve our energy and attitude by staying active and eating well.

I want you to take a few minutes to seriously consider these questions:

- Why can't you have tons of energy?
- Why can't you feel great about yourself?
- Why can't you be the picture of health?
- Why can't you be an example of health to your kids?
- Why can't you walk a 5K, run a 10K, or even run a marathon?
- Why can't you (fill in the blank)?

Why not you?

WHAT ARE YOUR GOALS?

"The greatest danger for most of us is not that our aim is too high and we miss it. Rather, it's that we aim too low and we reach it."
— Michelangelo

What are your fitness and weight-loss goals? What do you really want to accomplish? Try to allow your ideas to come up without any judgments. Have you ever dreamed of accomplishing something and then talked yourself out of it by saying something like "I could never do that!" If so, I want you to reconsider.

You can do anything you set your mind to—you just need to take small steps, avoid excuses, come up with a plan to pull it off, and then make it happen! Have you ever dreamed of walking or running a 5K, 10K, half marathon, or marathon? Is there a hike or a walking trail you've eyed for years but never got in shape enough to do? Have you dreamed of being at a certain goal weight, having limitless energy, and feeling truly amazing?

Many people's fitness and weight-loss dreams have faded because life has gotten insanely busy. But the following quote speaks to how you can recommit to your dreams and goals at any time and at any age:

"It is never too late to be what you thought you could have been!"
— Author Unknown

Please read the above quote three times and then think of what your biggest fitness and weight-loss goals have been. Why can't you become a 5K finisher or a marathon finisher? Why can't you be at your goal weight and have limitless energy? If you follow my lead each day the only answer or thought in response to reaching lofty goals is "Yes I can!"

Dreaming small doesn't do you any good! Dream big when it comes to your fitness and weight-loss goals. If you currently can't run for five minutes but used to love running when you were younger, you could state your dream as "I'm going to run a 10K (six miles) within six months!" Or if you want to really dream big, "I'm going to run (or walk) my first marathon within twelve months!" You can accomplish anything you set your mind to—you really can!

It's OK if your goals make you nervous! Your goals should be challenging enough that they scare you a little bit. If they don't scare you, then you're aiming too low! Or put another way from earlier in the book:

Have you ever accomplished anything great without being scared?

Once you've come up with your fitness and weight-loss goals, make them concrete by dialing in the specifics. For example goals such as "I want to lose twenty pounds within five months" or "I want to be able to walk a 20-minute mile within thirty days" are ten times more motivating then "I want to lose weight" or "I want to be able to walk a mile." Once you've dialed in the specifics of your goals, the next key step is to write them down. Goals that aren't written down are still dreams.

After you write your goals down, post them on your fridge. This announces to your family (and yourself) that you're serious this time and that you're going for it! Now is your time to aim high and get after it! You'll be shocked to see what you accomplish and who you become in the process.

FOUR WORDS THAT CHANGED MY LIFE

It was 1995, and I was sitting on the train in Boston heading home from my finance job (I was a financial analyst at Fidelity Investments). A guy who had just run the Boston Marathon was sitting next to me. He was all sweaty, and his energy (given that he had just run a marathon) was amazing and very contagious.

I asked in amazement: "Did you just run the marathon?"

He said, "Yes, and it was the most amazing thing I've ever done!" He proceeded to tell me about his magical experience.

At the end of our conversation, he said to me "You should do it!" It was a powerful moment that literally transformed my life.

I weighed 224 pounds (40 pounds more than I do today) and as you can imagine, was not exactly marathon ready. I had played soccer in college and was fit, but long work hours and poor nutrition had packed on the pounds. But I was so excited after seeing the look in this guy's eyes that I decided to run the Boston Marathon the following year. I actually called my dad that night to tell him the big news, and he was excited for me. That guy truly changed my life forever!

I ran my first Boston Marathon that next year (in 1996) and have now run every year since. I'm up to eighteen straight Boston Marathons at the time of the publishing of this book in 2013. More importantly, I've run seventeen straight years to raise funds for the Dana-Farber Cancer Institute, where my mom was treated for lung cancer when I was young. This is a big motivator for me personally and it illustrates the power of finding your why. I have now kept 40 pounds off for over 18 years!

The simple statement "you should do it" transformed my life.

I'm not telling you this story in an effort to turn you into a marathon runner or a runner at all. But I am telling you that "you should do it." What is "it"? You decide, but it has something to do with setting a big fitness or weight-loss goal (one that really scares you and instigates action) and then making it happen.

Maybe "it" is walking continuously for ten minutes. Maybe "it" is walking a mile. Maybe "it" is walking or running a 5K, a 10K, a half marathon, or a full marathon. The key is to set a firm goal and then get after it!

This one decision could change your life like the guy on the train in Boston in 1995 changed mine by saying, "You should do it!"

CHAPTER 5: UNSTOPPABLE

IDENTIFY YOUR STRONG "WHYS" THEN CRUSH IT

When you start a weight-loss program, it's important that you have strong "whys," or reasons that will motivate you to take action even when you don't want to. Losing weight to fit into a pair of jeans, to look good on vacation, or for your high school reunion isn't the kind of strong "why" that I'm talking about. In order to make permanent lifestyle changes, you need to have "whys" that are bigger in scope and focus on the issues in life that are truly important to you. It's OK if you want to look a certain way, and that will be a side benefit of your increase in health and fitness. In my experience, though, if that's your only reason or motivation for weight loss, then it most likely won't last, and you'll eventually put the weight back on.

Here are some examples of my powerful and compelling whys:

1) I want to be a healthy example to my kids. Our kids follow our lead: if we're sedentary and unhealthy, they're usually sedentary and unhealthy. And when we're active and healthy, they're usually active and healthy (now and in the future).
2) I want to live a long life and be around long enough to play with my great-grandkids.
3) I want to avoid diabetes, high blood pressure, heart disease, and certain cancers that often stem from obesity.
4) I don't want to die of cardiac arrest like my father, only meet one out of my nine grandkids, and be robbed of decades of memories with my kids and their families.

OK, those are my whys, now, I want you to grab a piece of paper and write down your strong "whys."

Here's some tough love: if you aren't willing to spend five minutes writing out why you want to lose weight and get fit, then you aren't ready to make your health a top priority. It's time to get ready, it's time to change your life, it's time to change your destiny, stop dreaming and establish real written goals. Stick with me and lets get this done! Go ahead, grab a pen and get to work!

WHEN CAN I MEET YOUR MOM?

One night when I was reading my son Benjamin (who was three at the time) a bedtime story, I mentioned my mom (I talk about her a lot to my sons Benjamin and Alexander). Benjamin replied, "When can I meet your mom?"

Sadly, when my mom was forty-six years old (and the mother of four), she was diagnosed with lung cancer and was given six months to live. She had always been great about showering us with love, and she'd already been an amazing mom. But when she got sick, she stopped sweating a lot of the details.

She didn't give up on what was important, but she refocused. She laughed more and stressed less. She held her hugs a bit longer. She didn't go crazy if the scale gave her a bad number. She enjoyed each day. She also compressed a life of lessons into two short years to set up me and my siblings to know what's important in life and how to handle ourselves.

My mom was a warrior and fought hard to beat cancer, but the disease took her life two years later at the young age of forty-eight—when I was twelve. She never got to meet any of her nine grandchildren. She never got to meet my wife, see Benjamin's smile, or play with Alexander.

When I got older and learned more about health and wellness, I realized that one of the reasons my mom was robbed of many amazing years was due to her unhealthy lifestyle. My mom was a smoker. She struggled with her weight. She was a single mother who worked three jobs to provide for her family. In all, she was so busy pouring herself into us, her children, that she didn't leave herself time to focus on her own health. She also didn't have the knowledge and the tools to get healthy.

Why am I pushing you to hold yourself accountable when it comes to your fitness and weight-loss goals? Because you deserve better than to be robbed of holding your grandkids someday! My mom deserved better, and you deserve better.

One year prior to my mom passing away, she wrote my three siblings and me a special letter. I'm sharing it with you here so that you can get a deep sense of purpose around why you deserve to lose weight, get fit, and hopefully avoid ever having to write a letter like this to your kids or family:

Please go to www.NoExcusesWorkouts.com/Book to read this powerful letter.

I've shared this with you in hopes that you'll grab hold of today and view it as a gift, that you'll add "Be a rock star grandparent or great-grandparent" to your list of "whys." Life is too short to sweat every detail. Each day is a gift. Stop putting off your dreams, and start making them happen today.

OUR KIDS BECOME US

One summer when I was getting ready for a run, my son Alexander (who was four years old at the time) said:

"Daddy, can I go running with you?"

I said sure, so prior to the actual run, Alexander joined me for the run that turned out to be my favorite run of 2012: a quick trip down the street and around our house.

Our kids become us! If we're active and eat healthfully, they'll mostly likely do the same. Unfortunately, the opposite is also true. According to the American Academy of Child and Adolescent Psychiatry:

- A child with one obese parent is 50 percent likely to become an obese adult.
- A child with two obese parents is 80 percent likely to become an obese adult.

As a parent, your weight and lifestyle have a significant impact on your child's activity level, eating habits, and outlook on weight.

Remember, being an example of health to your kids has nothing to do with your current weight, your jean size, or whether you're a runner. But it does have everything to do with how you live: whether you are active, watch your portions, stay hydrated and so on.

Set your kids up to be healthy adults by showing them the way now!

A SIX-YEAR-OLD'S SAD GOOD-BYE

On a recent flight I sat next to a wonderful woman named Joyce, who was probably in her mid-seventies and clearly upset.

When I asked her what was wrong, she told me that she was returning to Florida after attending her niece's husband's funeral. He was only forty-four years old.

Joyce was visibly sad as she recounted the experience of her recent trip: her niece had been talking with her husband just one week ago when he suddenly grabbed his chest and collapsed. He had suffered a heart attack, and the paramedics were unable to save him. The saddest part was that he had left behind a wonderful wife and a confused six-year old daughter.

Joyce explained to me how her nephew had been obese, had diabetes, and "did not pay attention to his health."

It broke my heart to hear this story because, as I shared earlier, I lost my own dad to cardiac arrest when I was twenty-three and he was just sixty-two). My dad was an amazing man who struggled with his weight most of his life, and his health suffered as a result. So I know firsthand what it feels like to lose a parent too early.

Unfortunately, most Americans don't pay attention to their health. They're too busy juggling the stresses of life—the kids, the house, the meals, the job—to eat right and exercise consistently.

But the sad thing is, if they were to improve their lifestyle and maintain a healthy weight, all the other important areas of their life would improve as well. They would have more energy to play with their kids, they would be more productive at work, they would be sick less, and most importantly they would be around for their loved ones.

It's a common belief that your weight only affects you, but that isn't true. Your health plays a pivotal role in the lives of the people around you: your friends, your loved ones, and your family. It's important to the people who love you that you're alive and healthy.

Please consider sharing this chapter with your spouse. If he or she is avoiding his or her health it's time to consider having an uncomfortable conversation about making positive changes. This will be one of the most important decisions of your life; don't miss this opportunity!

CHOOSE HOW TO SPEND YOUR GOLDEN YEARS

As I mentioned earlier, many people look at life as if they'll stay young forever. But the truth is we're all getting older. The key question to consider is this: How do you want to spend your golden years?

Do you want to have tons of energy and be able to go for long walks with your spouse? Do you want to be able to play golf and still work out? Do you want to be able to chase your grandkids or great-grandkids around the yard?

The simple and hard truth is that now is the time to form the habits and to become or stay healthy as you look toward your future. On a recent trip to the doctor's office, I thought it was very sad to see so many older people in very bad health. They were in wheelchairs and using oxygen machines, and many were very overweight. Please don't take this the wrong way—I'm not bringing it up to make you feel bad. I'm writing about it because I care about you and want to see you focus on your health and live a long, high-energy, and healthy life. Not only is this one of my strong "whys" but it is also what you deserve!

Since I truly believe that the actions we take now will lead to the things we're able to do when we're older, I always enjoy meeting people who've made healthy lifestyle choices and who are proof that these choices pay off later in life. The following are stories of some of the inspiring people I have met.

Carol

Carol is a very special person in my life. She was my mom's best friend. I was fortunate that after my mom passed away when I was twelve, Carol became like a mother to me. We're very close, and she has helped me tremendously throughout my life. She also happens to be an amazingly active woman for her age—seventy-five.

Carol does a strength training class two mornings per week, and she runs three miles three to four mornings per week. Carol took up running in her forties and says that she uses it to "stay sane." Isn't that great proof that it's never too late to start something new? She looks much younger than her age, and her positive energy and upbeat attitude are contagious.

How active are you going to be when you're seventy-five? Will you be able to walk or run three miles? Your actions today and over the years to come will either lead to your being sedentary (and dealing with health issues that may arise from that) or being a rock star when you're seventy-five.

I say you decide right now that you want to be like Carol on your seventy-fifth birthday!

Great Gramma Florence

My wife Karen's grandmother flies out to see us every year at Thanksgiving. We have always remarked on how much energy she has when she is with us. I remember that one particular year, when she was seventy-eight, we were amazed by her activity level. Alexander and Benjamin were little (three and one), and the first day with us, Great Gramma spent about five to six hours playing with them on the *floor*! She also chased Alex around the house and wore him out before she became tired herself. Since she has always played with the boys, they both describe her as "fun."

Most seventy-eight-year-olds (or even fifty-eight-year-olds) aren't able to get down on the floor and play with their grandkids or great-grandkids for hours. But that's how I'm planning on being when I'm a great-grandfather! How about you?

Eighty-Year-Old Esther

One day at the gym, I chose the treadmill next to an older woman I had never spoken to but had always been a fan of at the gym. I was there to do my intervals, but I was excited to also have an opportunity to learn more about this amazing woman.

After saying hello and talking a bit, I introduced myself. Here's what my new workout buddy said: "My name is Esther, and I'm eighty. I've done this every day for many years."

She was walking fast (I mean fast) on the treadmill. I told her she looked amazing, and she said "I've been active my whole life! I just do the best I can—I'm not in great shape." Meanwhile she honestly looked like should could run for miles if she wanted to. I then replied, "How many other eighty-year-olds do you know who are fit and look as good as you?"

Her reply really made me think: "I don't have many friends my age because they're all gone, or the few that are left aren't able to even walk on their own."

And then my new workout buddy started focusing on her workout again.

I want to be like Esther later in life: She is an eighty-year-old rock star.

Grandma Mary: Ninety-Three Years Old and Still Rocking

When Karen and I went to our friend David's fortieth birthday party, David's ninety-three-year-old grandmother was there. She was sitting on a couch drinking a beer (yes, I'm serious), and she fit in and was engaging in conversations perfectly. I was floored!

About thirty minutes later, Grandma Mary was sitting alone, so I went over and introduced myself. I said to her, "OK, I want to know your secret." She replied, "What secret?" I said, "How you look so good and are so on at ninety-three years old!" (She had shared her age during the early part of our discussion.)

Her answer: "I don't take any pills. None. I worked hard all my life. I stay active, and I watch what I eat."

I don't know about you, but I want to be just like Mary when I'm ninety-three. Her advice was so simple (note—not easy), yet highly effective. She is truly amazing!

TODAY'S ACTIONS DICTATE THE QUALITY AND NUMBER OF FUTURE HOLIDAYS

Most people don't think about how today's actions and overall lifestyle play such an important role in their future, including the length and quality of their lives. We are so busy rushing through our days that we don't realize our health is slipping away.

There are two options when it comes to aging:

1) Avoid making your health a priority and spend your golden years unhealthy, having no energy, taking pills that generally mask health issues versus curing them, and unable to do much. This approach most likely will limit not only the quality but also the actual length of your life. Scary, but true.
2) Make your health a top priority, stay active, watch what you eat, save a ton of money by not having to take many (or any) pills, and keep doing the things you've always loved to do (like going to birthday parties and having a beer)—and live a long and fun life!

The examples of the people I mentioned above all point to the fact that if you stay active and healthy, you can have a high quality of life when you're older. Could this be one of your important "whys"? It is definitely one of mine!

Whether your important "whys" are your family, your friends, living a long and healthy life, or anything else that speaks to you, these are the motivating factors that will keep you going through the hard times. These things will help you commit to your workouts and good nutrition, and to refocus when you need to get back on track. So identify your important "whys," and get ready to make your fitness and weight-loss goals reality.

CHAPTER 6: BURN THE BRIDGE BEHIND YOU

UNLOCK YOUR PERSONAL BRILLIANCE

The quote below is one of my favorites because it helps us shift into embracing how great we can be.

> "Our deepest fear is not that we are inadequate. Our deepest fear is that we are powerful beyond measure. It is our light, not our darkness, that most frightens us. We ask ourselves, who am I to be brilliant, gorgeous, talented, and fabulous?
> Actually, who are you not to be?
> You are a child of God. Your playing small doesn't serve the world. There's nothing enlightened about shrinking so that other people won't feel insecure around you.
> We are all meant to shine, as children do. We are born to make manifest the glory of God that is within us. It's not just in some of us, it's in everyone. And as we let our own light shine, we unconsciously give other people permission to do the same.

As we are liberated from our own fear, our
presence automatically liberates others."
— Marianne Williamson

This amazing quote speaks to the fact that each of us has potential we never dreamed of. Most of us (me included) are stuck in first, second, or third gear—not realizing that we have five gears and that we can do magical things if we let go of our fears and go after our dreams.

What dreams have you been afraid to attempt? You have been given amazing gifts; you just need to find the courage to use them!

FEAR OF FAILURE

"What would you attempt to do if you knew
you could not fail?"
— Author Unknown

I love this quote, and I have it in my office. As we discussed earlier, if you're afraid of failing when it comes to your fitness and weight-loss goals, you're normal. We're all fearful of failing, but don't let that keep you from taking action or being successful.

If you knew you wouldn't fail, what dreams would you chase down? How fit would you become? How much weight would you lose and keep off for the rest of your life?

Here's another important question that I presented to you earlier in the book: When was the last time you did something great without being scared? If you look back on your life, you'll realize you were scared during all of your biggest growth opportunities: getting married, having kids and more. Embrace the fear and conquer it!

Copy the above quote onto a piece of paper and put it where you'll see it every day. I have it right next to my computer in my office so that I see it often. Truly believe that you're not going to fail! You're going to be successful by taking small steps, following my lead, and taking it one decision and one day at a time!

FAILURE IS NOT AN OPTION

If you're like many people, you've attempted to lose weight and get fit before. You've tried gym memberships, diet pills, personal trainers, diets, infomercial products and other methods, with little or no success. An unfortunate outcome of some of these failed efforts is that sometimes you try the next thing almost looking for a reason to fail. You ask yourself: Will intervals really work? Does the No Excuses Workout truly work all my major muscle groups with no equipment? Am I going to be successful?

Earlier in the book we discussed focusing on reasons to win instead of reasons to fail. In addition to that new strategy, I want you to shift your thinking to "failure is not an option." Remember, failure means you have stopped trying and you've given up. However, overeating for a weekend or not working out for a few days doesn't mean you've failed. It means you've merely experienced a set-back. Take my advice and join me with a "failure is not an option" attitude. Remind yourself of this if you stumble or have a tough day or two, and reach out to me for support when the going gets tough. You are not alone!

When you approach our system with a "failure is not an option" outlook you won't give power to your negative voice. Just cut yourself off from the thought or option of failing so that you position yourself to do what it takes to be successful!

90% OF ALL FAILURE IS DUE TO QUITTING

Most of the time when people start an exercise program, they're probably very close to success when they quit. There are many reasons people quit and fail in their attempts to lose weight and get fit, but I think the number-one reason is attitude. If you remain positive, are realistic about results, roll with the punches (because things often go wrong), focus on long-term goals, and take it one day at a time, you're going to be successful!

On the other hand, if you're negative, make everything a big deal, and continuously get discouraged about workouts missed, weight not lost, overeating, etc., then you're set up for failure. You deserve to feel good about yourself, to have tons of energy, and to be healthy! So focus on having a positive attitude, and the next time your negative voice tries to drag you down and talk you into failing, fight back by focusing on staying positive—and remember that 90 percent of failure is due to quitting. Keep fighting and never give up—you're worth it.

BURN THE BRIDGE BEHIND YOU

I first learned about this concept from one of my Jim Rohn motivational CDs. "Burning the bridge behind you" is about deciding what you want, getting after it, and cutting yourself off from retreating. I want you to take this approach to your fitness and weight-loss journey. Enough is enough. You've been battling with getting fit and losing weight for far too long, and you deserve to reach your goals and stay there.

It's time (right now) to burn the bridge behind you, become the new, high-energy and healthy version of you that you know lies within you, and then never look back!

What would happen if you cut yourself off from the option of ever going back to the person you were before you lost weight and got in great shape? Think of being on an island prior to starting your wellness journey. Let's call it the "I'm tired of feeling terrible and having no energy" island. Now, you work hard-nailing your workouts, limiting your portion sizes, following my "Fifteen Secrets to Better Health" - to build a bridge to the "I have tons of energy, feel great about myself, and am healthy and happy" island.

All the clothes that no longer fit you (because you've gotten so fit) or are about to not fit you (because you're about to get so fit) need to be given to charity. That way your options are to stay fit or to walk around naked (or spend a lot of money on new clothes that you already had). This is what I mean by burning the bridge behind you. I want you to cut yourself off from the option of failure by leaving no chance to "go back." Is this scary? Yes. But it's also worth it because *you* are worth it! As I mentioned earlier, the greatest things we accomplish in life are usually scary...scary, but worth it.

You deserve to have tons of energy, to feel great about yourself, and to be healthy. So burn the bridge behind you, follow the Fifteen Secrets to Better Health and enjoy the new you!

CHAPTER 7:
CRANK UP YOUR ENERGY

WHAT'S YOUR ENERGY LEVEL?

How much energy do you have? Are you generally upbeat and feel like you could go all day, or are you dragging through your afternoon drinking one soda after the next? Now compare how many workouts you're doing per week with how much energy you have.

The amount of exercise you do has a *huge* impact on your energy levels! Yes, when you first start an exercise program, you might feel exhausted for a week or two. But once you get through that initial phase, you draw tremendous positive energy from your workouts and from staying fit.

If you say to yourself that you don't have the energy to exercise today, please consider changing that thinking to "I need to exercise today in order to boost my energy."

On a scale of one to five (one means you are dragging and five means you are on fire and are jumping out of your skin), what is your energy level?

Starting today, focus on improving your energy by exercising, watching what you eat, and making healthy choices. The time you invest in these efforts will pay off in many ways (especially with huge increases in energy) and is worth every minute of sweat.

REAL ENERGY VERSUS FAKE ENERGY

Where are you getting your energy?

There are two kinds of energy:

1) Real energy that is produced by sleeping well, eating right, and exercising.
2) Fake energy that is produced by consuming coffee, soda, energy drinks, and sugar-laden junk food.

We each make an important series of decisions each day: Where am I going to get the energy I need to power through my day?

Where do you get energy each day? Honestly, think about this for a minute or two. Option two, or getting energy from caffeine and/or sugar, hurts your health and feeds your lack of fitness and weight-loss results. Option one, or getting energy from more natural sources, like rest and exercise, fuels your fitness and weight-loss results and expedites the time between now and your becoming who you deserve to be.

Where are you getting your energy today?

HAVING LOW ENERGY IS ZERO FUN

Sometimes when I'm focused on a special project for work, I end up working late into the night. One particular night, I was up until 2:00 a.m. working and then had to get up with my son Alexander at 5:30 a.m. since my wife, Karen, was sick. After a total of three hours and thirty minutes of sleep (I usually get seven hours), I was really hurting on Friday (and even into Saturday).

On Friday my energy level was at about a one on a scale of one to five (five being the best). I drank much more coffee than usual and even bought a soda in the afternoon, as I was dragging. I couldn't help but think about the fact that many people spend all their days dragging and having no or low energy. And it's not a fun way to live!

Going through this gave me a taste of what many people deal with very day.

When you have low energy, you aren't excited about your job (either at an office or doing the hardest job on the planet—being a Mom). And you don't have the energy that your kids are expecting every time they want to play with you.

Life is too short to spend with low energy. You deserve more and should aim for being a five on the energy scale. Wouldn't it feel great to jump out of bed each morning with lots of energy? It *is* possible to feel this way. You just need to focus on getting enough rest, eating healthy, and getting plenty of exercise.

FOCUS ON YOUR ENERGY AND HEALTH, NOT YOUR WEIGHT!

I want you to start focusing on cranking up your energy and improving your health, and forget about focusing on weight loss. When you focus on being healthy - fitting in your workouts, drinking your water, not skipping meals and only having dessert once a week - the weight loss takes care of itself.

I'm not telling you to stop weighing yourself once a week (which is my normal recommendation).

I'm telling you that focusing on your weight alone will drive you crazy. If you focus on increasing your energy and improving your health by following my lead, I'm confident you'll lose a healthy, realistic, and sustainable 1 to 3 pounds per week (or 52 to 156 pounds in one year).

Instead of focusing only on weight loss, look at the choices you make each day as opportunities to crank up your energy and mood and improve your health! If you increase your water intake, eat every two to three hours, watch your portion sizes and park in the farthest spot at the grocery store, you will have more energy, and you will lose weight. You will be amazed by how much switching your focus improves your results and how much more fun getting in shape will be.

GET ENERGY FROM EXERCISE

As just mentioned you can significantly increase your energy through exercise. In fact, I think the best reward for staying consistent with your workouts is the earned increase in energy level. Yes, fitting into smaller jeans or losing weight is nice. But feeling like you have enough energy to jump through the roof is the real reward.

I do have one caveat: when you start an exercise program, you might have less energy than usual. This is simply because your body needs to adapt to having to work harder than it is used to. But don't let the one to two weeks that this can take force you to associate exercise with robbing yourself of energy. Look at it like taking two steps back to eventually take ten forward.

If you don't start feeling like you have more energy from your new habit of consistent exercise after about two weeks, then please consider the following:

1) Are you doing too much (too many workouts and/or exercising too hard or long)?
2) Are you sleeping enough?
3) Are you eating enough calories and staying hydrated throughout the day?

You deserve to have tons of energy and to feel great, so concentrate on being consistent with your workouts, and you'll be amazed by how much more energy you will have.

THE #1 WAY TO REDUCE STRESS

Exercise is the quickest, cheapest, and simplest way to reduce stress. In fact, the more stressed you are, the more you should focus on nailing your workouts. Even though you may not feel up to a workout, think of it as an investment in your health. Remember, when you finish each workout you are a better person than when you started. You will feel ten times better, have more energy, have higher self-esteem, and are always in a better mood!

Even a five-minute walk can clear your head and make you feel better, so make exercise your number-one tool in fighting stress. You and your health are worth it!

ARE YOU IRRITABLE DUE TO LACK OF EXERCISE?

Like most people I have times when I'm honestly too busy to fit in my normal workouts. As you can imagine, I don't like it when I'm unable to work out, and one reason is because during these times I become irritable.

Do you get irritable when you don't exercise regularly? You may not realize it, but you probably do. The sad thing is, not only do you not feel good about yourself and feel off when you don't exercise, but your family and those around you have to suffer the consequences of your being irritable and not at your best.

Instead of looking at exercise as something you have to do to lose weight, look at it as your attitude adjuster and the number-one way to feel better!

Again, if you don't count on exercise as a cure for stress, it's time to put it to the test. Take it from me it works every time!

ENTER YOUR NEW YOU PHONE BOOTH

As I walked across the gym parking lot one day after nailing my interval workout, I was thinking how I literally felt ten times better than I had felt walking into the gym. I then started thinking about how Clark Kent would jump into a phone booth and come out a new person: Superman!

As I have said, the person who finishes a workout is always a much more energetic, positive, and happy person than the one who started it. So, if you know you have a "new you phone booth" available to you every day, then why do you only enter it a few times per week or not at all?

Instead of looking at your workouts as burdens to check off your crazy schedule, look at them as energy and mood boosters!

SEVENTY-SEVEN TO THIRTY

I saw my friend Jim (who is now seventy-seven years young) at the fitness club after one of his daily swims. He was glowing and was in his usual positive spirits, and when I asked him how his swim was he said:

"I feel seventy-seven years old when I start and thirty when I finish!" Then he added, "There's no medication on this planet that give me what I get out of my exercise."

Wow! Think about this for a minute. There is no better way to beat the aging process and no better way to lift your spirits, energy, and mood than exercise.

SWEATING TO FEEL GREAT

Can I share a secret with you? There's something powerful and empowering about sweating. It tells you that you're working hard enough and lets you know you're getting the most out of your workout. I see a lot of people at the gym doing cardio, and yet they're either not sweating or are barely sweating at all. That's a missed opportunity. And the unfortunate thing is, many of them will eventually quit on themselves and their workouts because they are "not getting results" even though they're putting in the time.

Solution: Learn to love sweat! Hey, it actually feels good. Sweat is your reward for working hard. It shows that you're working at a moderate to high intensity and therefore are maximizing your fitness and weight-loss results. Although any movement (whether you're sweating or not) is great for your health, you might as well maximize your results while working out, so sweating is the way to go! Don't you want to get faster results? Trust me - work up a sweat!

If you've been given the OK from your doctor to exercise at moderate to high intensity and you've taken a week to start slowly, then you should definitely be sweating while exercising by the end of your second week. So get sweating, wear it proudly, and have fun!

LIFE IS BETTER WHEN YOU'RE FIT

When was the last time you were really fit? Honestly, think about it for a minute. Was it last year, before your first child was born, in college, or in high school? Think back to how much energy you had and how great you felt. Staying consistent with your workouts and eating well will lead to weight loss and your body changing, but the true benefit is the amazing feeling of being fit—having limitless energy and feeling healthy!

When you're fit, the little things are not a big deal; you smile more, are in a better mood, and definitely give off better energy to your kids, spouse, friends, and co-workers. You have a heightened level of self-confidence and you feel "on." If a friend calls and asks you to go for a walk or a hike, you're in! If you go to the mall and you want to try on some new jeans or a new bathing suit, it's not stressful—it's fun.

You don't have to get stressed about the weight you meant to lose or diets that crashed or workouts you've missed. You have the peace of mind of a job well done: you are fit and either at your goal weight or inching closer each day.

If you don't already feel amazing, then I invite you to make you and your health a top priority so that you realize how much better life is when you feel great and are fit. You are worth it!

3 OUT OF 168 WILL CHANGE YOUR LIFE

There are 168 hours per week, and we all are all given a clean slate of these hours every week.

The people who accomplish amazing things in life (including hitting their goal weight, getting fit, and staying there) make the important decision to allocate a certain amount of time to exercise.

Please honestly add up the hours you spend each week doing the following:

1) watching TV
2) using the Internet (for entertainment)
3) exercising

The average American spends 4.5 hours per day watching TV (that's 31.5 hours per week)!

If you commit to spending three hours out of the 168 hours you have available each week (that's six days of working out thirty minutes per day), then you will be shocked by how much your entire life will improve!

You deserve to have tons of energy and to thrive, and three consistent hours of exercise per week is all you need to get there. Make the decision right now that you and your health are worth it and commit to my 3 out of 168 challenge.

CHAPTER 8: CHASE PROGRESS, NOT PERFECTION

PERFECTION OR SUCCESS: IT'S YOUR CHOICE

If you try to be perfect with your workouts or your eating, you will constantly let yourself down, and your negative voice will eventually talk you into quitting. No one is perfect, so why would you try to hold yourself to that standard? Release the stress associated with trying to be perfect, and instead start focusing your energy on chasing progress.

To be successful in getting fit and losing weight, you have to hold yourself accountable and take action. But you also have to be a realist and recognize that you cannot do everything perfectly. Some days you may not have time to do a full workout. Taking steps like doing a six-minute No Excuses Workout because you don't have the time to do the full twenty-four minutes are victories worth celebrating. No, it's not perfect, but it keeps you "in the game."

Some weeks you will crush it and lose one to three pounds, and other weeks you will stumble and not see great results. But as long as you're making progress overall, you'll get to your goal weight!

Instead of chasing perfection, focus 100 percent of your energy on being persistent and making your health a top priority. Perfection is unattainable, and letting go of this pipe dream will free you to become the high-energy and healthy version of yourself that you deserve to be.

TOXIC PERFECTIONISM

If you're having trouble letting go of perfectionism, then please grab a pen and a piece of paper and answer the following questions:

Question # 1: Do you expect perfection of yourself as far as your workouts? If so, how has this served you in the past as far as your efforts to get fit and lose weight?

Question #2: Do you expect perfection of yourself as far as your nutrition? If so, how has this served you in the past as far as your efforts to get fit and lose weight?

Question #3: Do you tend to quit fitness and weight-loss programs because you give up once you realize you haven't done it perfectly?

Question #4: (a tough but very important question for parents): Do you think it's healthy for your kids to learn perfectionism from you? Do you think they will be at a disadvantage as adults if they are perfectionists?

Question #5: Have you ever attempted to lose weight and get fit by focusing on just doing the best you can and ditching the toxic idea of being perfect?

Think of what you would write to your best friend if she or he were trying to ditch perfectionism then write yourself a note telling yourself why you deserve the freedom of ditching perfectionism and what that will do for your energy, mood, weight, health, happiness, and family!

HOW DO YOU DEFINE SUCCESS?

Many people define success as reaching a weight-loss goal. But could success be defined as incorporating new, healthy habits into your life? Once you've done that then the results (more energy, good health and weight loss) will take care of themselves.

Instead of judging whether you are successful by looking at the scale, focus on building consistent, healthy habits.

7 TIPS TO DITCH ALL-OR-NOTHING THINKING

Just as it's important not to expect perfection when it comes to fitness and weight loss, it's also important to avoid engaging in all-or-nothing thinking. How many times have you splurged on your diet or skipped a few workouts and then completely given up on your fitness routine? Making a couple of mistakes doesn't mean that all is lost. By ditching all-or-nothing thinking, you can experience a few speed bumps and still continue on the same path.

Here are my seven tips to ditch all-or-nothing thinking:

1) **Be aware that the negative voice in your head** will push you towards an all-or-nothing approach to your fitness and weight-loss. When you have that

voice, tell yourself "I'm better than that". Stay positive and keep moving.

2) **Missing workouts or occasionally eating badly only means you are human.** Just because you slipped up doesn't mean you need to give up. Each day is a new day to be healthy, so jump back in the game and forget about yesterday.
3) **Focus on winning today** and then repeat it again tomorrow. You don't have to worry about how much weight you have to lose or how many workouts you need to do. All you need to do is focus on taking one day at a time!
4) **Redefine what a workout is.** Here is my definition: anything that gets your heart rate up and works your muscles more than when your sitting down.
5) **Do Random Acts of Fitness** by turning everyday activities into workouts. Park far from the door at the store or office, march in place while brushing your teeth, or put one piece of clothing away at a time while doing laundry. Be creative - it really adds up!
6) **Eat a healthy breakfast within one hour of waking up** every morning to set a healthy nutritional tone for the day.
7) **Drink water all day long** by carrying a water bottle. This helps you stay hydrated and is great for your overall health.

You deserve to have tons of energy and to feel great, so focus on these seven tips, and you should be able to ditch the all-or-nothing approach to your fitness and weight-loss journey.

CHAPTER 9:
IDENTIFY YOUR RESULTS ROBBERS

HOW TO AVOID THE TOP 6 RESULTS ROBBERS

There are probably three to six habits that are 90 percent of the problem as far as your cracking the code on losing weight and getting fit. These are what I like to call Results Robbers. Once you identify the ones that are costing you the most, you can focus on avoiding them and then watch your results take off.

Here are the top six Results Robbers and how to avoid them:

1) Having dessert five to seven nights per week:

Many people, including me, have a sweet tooth. My approach to nutrition is not about denying yourself the foods you like but instead eating them in moderation. Instead of having a high-calorie dessert every night, limit that special treat to one night per week. On the other days it's OK to eat something sweet, but choose something healthy and with less calories than your dessert of the week.

Are you ready to make the magic happen, then lets do the math together: When you substitute a 100-calorie yogurt for your daily 500-calorie dessert you save 400 calories per day. Now, focus on having that 500-calorie dessert only one day per week. You will consume 2,400 less calories per week or 124,800 less calories per year. That is staggering! Since you have to burn 3,500 calories more than you consume to lose one pound, just making this one important change will help *you lose approximately thirty-six pounds in one year!* If you don't believe me, take out your calculator and do the math! If you are feeling hopeful right now, you should be!

2) Not eating frequently enough:

The frequency of your meals is as important as the quality of what you eat. If you skip breakfast or don't eat it within one hour of waking up, this slows down your metabolism. If you don't eat every two to three hours, you end up coming into your two major meals (lunch and dinner) very hungry, and this causes you to make bad choices and to overeat. So eat breakfast within an hour of waking up, and then eat healthy midmorning and midafternoon snacks to keep your metabolism cranking throughout the day.

3) Taking weekends off from exercising and eating right:

Your weekends (Friday evening through Monday morning) represent one-third of your week. So if you eat badly and blow off your workouts all weekend, you cancel out all of your hard work from the rest of the week. Life's too short to spin your wheels and not achieve fitness and weight-loss results, especially if you're making healthy food choices and nailing your workouts during the week.

You don't have to worry about every detail on the weekends, but you should wear your "everything in moderation" hat. You can have a few glasses of wine or a few beers and enjoy some of your favorite foods, just don't over-do it. And make sure to do at least one workout over the weekend. Follow this approach and you will start the next week ready to go!

4) Not taking 100 percent ownership of your health:

Are you holding yourself accountable when it comes to your workouts and your eating habits? Be honest—are you?

If you're going to continue to let yourself make excuses for skipping workouts, eating seconds and having that second glass of wine, then reaching your fitness and weight-loss goals is either going to take a very long time or it's never going to happen. You want the truth, so I am giving it to you!

Hold yourself accountable for the workout goals you've set. If you've stated (and hopefully written down) that you're going to do three Interval Workouts and two No Excuses Workouts per week, you should be holding yourself accountable and making the workouts happen.

Please take a few minutes to really think about this. It's extremely important. No one else is going to make you accountable for staying consistent. You need to take control and be firm with yourself about your own accountability. Yes, staying consistent with your workouts and eating well is actually do what it takes to get results and claim the victory you deserve!

5) **Telling yourself "I don't have time" to exercise while spending time watching TV or online each day:**

How much time do you spend watching TV and online each day, and how much time do you spend exercising each day?

Honestly, if you haven't done this already, please grab a piece of paper and come up with an average day. Remember, playing with your kids, washing your windows, and doing other things that get your heart rate up should be included as part of your exercise time.

If you're watching TV and spending time online during the day or evening and you say you don't have time to exercise, then you might as well be saying "My health is not important to me!" Lying to ourselves about not having time to exercise is a key reason most people don't achieve their fitness and weight-loss goals.

If this is one of your Results Robbers, fit it and reward yourself with time watching TV or online only after you have done at least 10 minutes of exercise.

6) **Having an all-or-nothing approach to fitness and weight loss:**

   As we talked about earlier, perfectionism will keep you from ever reaching your potential. We all make mistakes. There will always be speed bumps in the road. All you have to do is to keep moving over those speed bumps and before long you will be coasting toward your goals!

How many of these Results Robbers have robbed you of fitness and weight-loss results? Life's too short to not feel good about yourself and not have tons of energy, so focus on stopping these six Results Robbers, and your rocket will leave the pad.

ARE YOU AVOIDING THE SCALE?

Another major Results Robber is avoiding the scale. We receive e-mails from No Excuses system members about once a week asking us to change their starting weight. They enter an amount while registering (they usually guess) and then e-mail us to have our software team change the number, after they actually weigh themselves.

On average the actual amount is usually around ten pounds higher than the member thought.

You can't figure out where you're going unless you know where you are right now. I realize this is an uncomfortable subject for many people, but I want you to weigh yourself right now because I care about you, and I know it will help motivate you to improve your health.

This will give you facts you can work with, and it's the initial motivation for you to make today your January 1st and to get moving. Grab a pen right now and write down your weight and today's date:

Your Actual Weight: ___________
Today's Date: ___________

Here is something fun to think about. You are going to come back to this page in a few months and smile at how far you have come!

Although I talk in my daily e-mails and my weekly radio shows about not focusing all of your energy on your weight, it is an important number for you to track. We're focusing on improving your health, increasing your energy, improving your self-esteem, and making you an example of health to your kids, but we can't risk avoiding your weight.

I suggest that you weigh yourself once a week and take your measurements once per month. I weigh myself every Monday morning and have for many years. Although I have kept over forty pounds off for over eighteen years, I still do this to make sure I'm cranking along.

Remember when weighing yourself that while it's good to have this information, it's only a number.

Weighing yourself every day is not a good idea because most people either have a good or bad day based on what the scale says. Plus (and more importantly), so many things play into your weight on a daily basis (sleep, nutrition, hydration, menstrual cycles, stress, etc.) that you really can't see trends by weighing yourself every day. On the other hand, weighing yourself every week will give you the big picture.

Some weeks you will lose one to three pounds and other weeks you may gain one or two pounds. In fact, when you start doing strength training (like the No Excuses Workout), you could actually gain weight because muscle is denser than fat. Replacing fat with muscle could lead to a small increase in weight. The key is to not get discouraged and to continue focusing on your health. If you have more energy and your pants are looser, you're moving in the right direction. If you continue to focus on following my lead, not only will you feel better but the weight loss will take care of itself.

WHAT'S YOUR TARGET WEIGHT?

Yet another Results Robber is setting unrealistic weight-loss goals for yourself. If you focus on these often-unattainable goals, you'll never be satisfied with your results. This is why I encourage people to focus on feeling healthy, having more energy, losing inches, and fitting more comfortably into their clothes, rather than focusing on a specific number on the scale. Yes, your weight can provide some important information, but it can also hinder your progress if you become too focused on it.

However, I do want to mention something very important: aim for your waist being equal to or less than half of your height in inches. So if you're five feet six (sixty-six inches tall), your waist ideally will be thirty-three inches or less. This is because your risk of developing heart disease, diabetes, high blood pressure, and many cancers goes up exponentially when your waist is larger than half of your height in inches.

BE HONEST ABOUT YOUR RESULTS

As you start and then move forward on your fitness and weight loss journey be honest and ask yourself if you're seeing and feeling results. This is a good time to re-visit the 15 Secrets and to ask yourself honestly how much time you have spent evaluating and implementing them. Here are some good questions to ask yourself that will give you additional information beyond the number you see on the scale:

- Do you have more energy?
- Are your clothes getting loose and/or are you losing inches off your body?
- Do you feel better about yourself?
- Do you feel healthier?
- Are your muscles more defined or toned?
- Are you getting your negative voice to zip it?

If you aren't achieving results, then it's time to be honest with yourself and change your approach. Even changing small things can make a big difference over time.

I've been going to the same gym for many years, and most of the members look the same as they did when I joined. The sad part is that many of them are at the gym a lot. But I only see about one out of every twenty people in the cardio area doing Interval Workouts and more than half of the people are barely sweating. I also see a lot of people standing around while doing strength training and not paying attention to their form.

If you've been consistent with your workouts and aren't seeing positive changes in your body, then it's time to refocus and change what you're doing. I love the following quote:

> "The definition of insanity is doing the same thing over and over and expecting different results."
> — Albert Einstein

Life's too short to be exercising and not seeing results. If you're putting in the time to exercise, you deserve results. If you aren't putting in the time, then reading this book will help you stop making excuses and recommit so you're on the right path!

TAKE 100% OWNERSHIP OF YOUR WEIGHT

"My will shall shape my future. Whether I fail or succeed shall be no man's doing but my own. I am the force; I can clear any obstacle before me, or I can be lost in the maze. My choice, my responsibility, win or lose, only I hold the key to my destiny."
— Elaine Maxwell

People often blame others and things (family, genes, lack of money and lack of time) for why they're overweight or out of shape. This is simply not true.

Your weight and fitness level are 100 percent yours to own. You can't blame anyone else; you need to take ownership and then take action! Acting on this one tip is probably the most important thing you will learn in this book.

As soon as you stop trying to pin the blame on others, you move into the driver's seat to make the changes to your daily habits that take you in the direction of your fitness and weight-loss goals. I know there is a high-energy and healthy version of you that is inside and ready to be revealed.

Once you take 100 percent ownership, your rocket will leave the pad and you'll shock yourself with what you accomplish and who you become. Now is your time to own it and then crush it!

STOP MAKING EXCUSES

Yet another Results Robber is making excuses. The more excuses you make (I don't have time to exercise, there's nothing healthy to eat, I don't have a gym membership and so on), the more your results decrease. The more results you achieve (increasing your energy, improving your health and losing one, two or even three pounds per week), the more your excuses decrease.

What's the relationship between making excuses and getting results? Honestly, think about this for a minute. They are inversely related—one goes up and the other goes down! Now is a great time to be candid with yourself about how excuses are affecting your fitness and weight-loss results.

Are you making excuses for why you can't fit in your workouts and eat right? If so, I want you to take a few minutes right now to think about the excuses you use to talk yourself out of maximizing your fitness and weight-loss results.

If you've used the "I don't have time to exercise" excuse, then I want you to look at how much time you spend online and watching TV each day and then be honest with yourself that it's not that you don't have the time to exercise.

If you've used the "there's nothing healthy to eat" excuse, I want you to think about how you can better prepare healthy options in the future.

If you've used the "I don't have a gym membership" excuse, I want you to focus on using this program, which does not require any time at the gym. Hopefully you have already gone through the 15 Secrets and seen that it includes links to a bunch of free workouts you can do right in your living room.

You deserve (not "need," not "should"—*deserve*) to stop making excuses and recommit to your workouts and healthy eating—starting right now.

No Excuses!

THE "BAD GENES" EXCUSE

Recently I saw a guy I'd met in the gym locker room three years ago, and he looks exactly the same as the day I met him. When we first met he asked me what I did, so

I told him how I am fortunate enough to spend my time guiding people in getting fit and losing weight.

He needs to lose about seventy-five pounds, and he said while explaining his current situation, "My problem is I have really bad genes." Saying that you have bad genes is an excuse to not take control of your health. I'm not denying that genes play a role in our health, but it's important not to use that as an excuse. Both of my parents struggled with their weight, especially my dad, but I have managed to break that cycle. You are better than using "your bad genes" as an excuse and I am living proof!

YOU'RE BETTER THAN THAT

The next time the negative voice in your head is trying to talk you into blowing off a workout or getting seconds or having your second, third, or seventh dessert of the week, I want you to say this to yourself:

You're better than that!

I love this saying because it's true and because it can help you during important decision-making moments when you're about to take a step in the wrong direction. Maybe "you're better than that" doesn't need to be your saying, but I do suggest you come up with something powerful to say to yourself. The point is to jolt you into really thinking about your health and how your daily decisions add up to victory or defeat on your journey.

Remember, you're better than that!

RESULTS COME FROM EFFORT

I was listening to one of my favorite Jim Rohn motivational CDs, and he said two very important statements that I want to share with you and I want you to think about:

- Finding is reserved for searchers.
- Reaping is reserved for sowers.

The fitness and weight-loss results you have and are going to achieve are complements of the effort you put forward. You don't get results without earning them! Are you putting in the effort needed to lose one to three pounds per week and to get in the best shape of your life? Only you know the answer. If not, take a look at your Results Robbers, make changes to fix them, and make results happen starting today. No excuses!

ALIGN YOUR CORE VALUES WITH YOUR ACTIONS

A big part of the frustration associated with not being at a healthy weight is the fact that the fitness and weight-loss areas of your life are contrasting against your core values.

What are your core values?

Even if you haven't considered this question in a while (or ever), you already have a set of core values that you live by. My top three are family, energy, and health.

Once you clearly identify your top three core values, you may see that in almost every area of your life (besides fitness and weight loss), you're in alignment with them. Part of the emotional exhaustion associated with not being able to lose weight is the subconscious misalignment of your core values and your actions.

Turn this negative into a source of strength and guidance by clearly identifying and writing down your top three core values. Then consider these values as you work hard to win the mental game (the true battleground) while losing weight and getting fit.

When your nutrition, exercise, and health-related decisions contradict your core values, call yourself out on it with power statements like "you're better than that!"

You will be pleasantly surprised how mentally freeing it is to have your new athletic lifestyle align with your core values. Embrace the power of this idea: You are an Athlete! You are Unstoppable!

CHAPTER 10:
TURN YOUR MIND INTO A POWER-FUL TOOL (NOT YOUR ENEMY)

EXERCISE AND NUTRITION ARE ONLY HALF OF WHAT LEADS TO SUCCESS

Yes, what exercise you do or what you eat is important as far as getting fit and losing weight. But if your head isn't in the right place, you'll never get and stay fit or lose weight for good! I believe that your attitude is 50 percent of what dictates your success, and I would place exercise at 25 percent and nutrition at 25 percent This is why approximately 50 percent of this book is focused on helping you shift your thinking so that you can build the mental muscles to be successful for good.

Here are a few key areas that are at the core of having the positive attitude you need to thrive:

- Being grateful for being healthy enough to walk
- Ditching all-or-nothing thinking
- Believing you are worth investing your time and energy into
- Avoiding the temptation of quick fixes
- Taking 100 percent ownership of your weight loss and fitness

When you have the mental muscles built and the healthy habits in place, you will free yourself to stay fit and lose weight for good. You will truly be unstoppable!

YOUR THOUGHTS DICTATE YOUR SUCCESS OR FAILURE

What do you think about? Honestly consider this for a few minutes. What do you think about most of the time? Are you generally thinking positive or negative thoughts about yourself, your circumstances, and your life?

If you are usually thinking negative thoughts or are negative in general, then that's probably going to pave the way to an uphill battle when it comes to your fitness and weight-loss goals.

If you're usually thinking positive thoughts or are positive in general, then that's probably going to pave your way to success. This is because you'll be able to roll with the punches when things go wrong; you won't beat yourself up over a few bad choices or days, and you'll be positive and grateful for being healthy enough to even walk.

Focus on staying positive, and I'm confident that you will shock yourself with your fitness and weight-loss results.

YOUR NEGATIVE VOICE VERSUS YOUR POSITIVE VOICE

Each day there is a pivotal battle that takes place in your head between your negative voice and your positive voice. Honestly think about these questions and your answers for a few minutes:

- Have you spent most of your life letting your negative voice run the show?
- Who would you be today if you had been listening to your positive voice all along?
- How much would you weigh today and how fit would you be if you had been listening to your positive voice for the last year?
- Why is it OK that your positive voice can barely be heard (or has been stuck in the basement for years)?

- Why do you let your negative voice convince you that you won't be able to get fit?
- How many attempts at losing weight and getting fit has your negative voice talked you out of in your life?

Your negative voice will even try to convince you that your current mental approach to weight loss is fine and that it's all about workouts and nutrition. But that is not the truth! In order to be successful on your weight-loss journey, you're going to have to learn how to get past some of your mental roadblocks, one of them being your negative voice.

At some point we all have a negative voice in our head telling us we can't finish a workout—or some other negative thought. Maybe you haven't exercised in a long time, and when you try to start the voice says, "You have too far to go—don't bother." Or when you're doing your interval workout and the final interval is challenging, the voice says, "You're too tired—blow it off." The key to being successful for the long haul with your fitness and weight-loss journey is to stay positive, ignore the negative voice, and keep fighting.

Remember, life's too short to beat yourself up over the weight you've gained, workouts you've missed, or eating badly for a day or two. All you can do is keep going and keep moving. Beating yourself up or listening to the negative voice in your head is only going to drag you in the wrong direction.

QUIET YOUR NEGATIVE VOICE

Here's a fact: it's difficult to get rid of your negative voice. Instead of having unrealistic expectations of losing the voice for good, embrace the fact that *you* are in control of the volume button for both your negative and positive voices.

People who are able to successfully lose weight and get in amazing shape have mastered the ability to control which voice they listen to! They turn down the volume on their negative voice and they crank up the volume on their positive voice.

From this point on, make a conscious effort to be fully aware of the internal debate between your negative and positive voices. This is the first step in getting ready to consistently invite your positive voice to the podium. Once you become more aware of your negative and positive voices, you can focus on controlling this process.

You can think of your negative voice as a bully who says mean things to you, makes you feel bad about yourself, and makes you afraid to do or try certain things. I have an example from my childhood that may help. Pretend you are confronting your bully as you listen to this story:

Chad was a mean kid who used to bully my brother Chris and I when we were kids. He would steal our lunches and say mean things. This went on until Chris decided enough was enough one day and stood up to Chad. Chad approached my brother with his usual barrage of mean comments and for the first time Chris did not back down and actually got in Chad's face. Once Chad realized that Chris was seriously not going to back down Chad left him alone and never bothered us again. Most bullies fold when someone actually stands up against them.

Your negative voice has been bullying you for far too long. It's time to stand up to that voice and start enjoying a judgment-free mind.

Here's how you can take down your bully: tell your negative voice that you aren't going to fail like you have in other attempts to lose weight and get fit. This time you're going to be successful because you're balancing smart nutrition and high-quality and quick workouts! Plus this approach is different because you're going to be aware of how often your negative voice is constantly trying to talk you down. Just as my older brother stood up to Chad, I am standing up for you.

At first, maybe your bully won't turn and run like Chad did when Chris finally confronted him. But your negative voice is going to run and hide as you lose weight keep it off for good! You've got the support you need and a proven system and it's time to claim victory at last!

Think about the following statement for a few minutes:

Your negative voice has robbed you and your family of too many victories!

If you're struggling to walk to the mailbox or struggling to finish your thirty-minute interval workout, don't let your negative voice drag you down. You're better than that, and you deserve to feel great about yourself and to have tons of energy!

DON'T JUDGE YOURSELF BASED ON WEIGHT

Does your weight really reflect who you are as a person? Of course not! It's just a number. It doesn't matter is you weigh five hundred pounds: you should never talk down to yourself or think negatively about yourself because of your weight—*ever*! I mean that.

No one is perfect—not you, not me—no one in this world.

Beating yourself up because you're overweight is only going to drag you in the wrong direction. Instead, focus on staying positive and making healthy choices. If you are making healthy choices, being consistent with your workouts and following my lead, then you are doing great and you should be proud of yourself—whether you weigh 500 pounds or 150 pounds.

I want you to throw your rearview mirror out the side of the car window. Yesterday is yesterday, and you can't do anything to change that. What you can do is embrace today and tomorrow, make healthy choices, avoid making excuses, and stay positive!

LOVE YOUR BODY

Yes, I'm serious. Your body is a gift, and you should love it. Regardless of whether you have one hundred pounds to lose or ten pounds to lose, you should cherish and love your body.

Your body and your health are true gifts. Yes, in an ideal world you would be at your goal weight and would love the way you look and would do the things you want to do. In the real world, however, life is hectic and challenging, so waiting until you achieve that perfect ideal to love your body is going to be a very long wait.

I want you to love your body and accept it for what it is (not how it looks). Loving your body is part of loving yourself. This concept can be challenging, since it's easy to compartmentalize what we love about ourselves.

For example, we love our laugh but not our thighs. We love our generosity but not our stomach. I invite you to love *all* of you, including all of your body...even the parts that aren't "perfect."

Taking this attitude will not only make you feel better about yourself overall, but it will also increase your motivation for sticking with this program. It's so much easier to take care of things we love.

The fact that you're this far into the book is a good sign. I know it, you should to. It means that you really do care about yourself and that you're committed to caring for the body you have. Embrace this fact and use it as motivation to continue on your journey.

THE POWER OF A POSITIVE ATTITUDE

A positive attitude is the number-one factor in determining whether you will be successful in losing weight and getting fit. Hey, bad things happen: the weather is terrible, your boss is being a nightmare, you oversleep, you skip your workout, your kids are sick and on and on it goes. One of the keys to true happiness is staying positive in the face of challenging situations. Lets be realistic, this is tough to do.

However, if you will open your mind and stay with me, you'll see how this will make a huge difference in how you feel and the vibe you give off to your family, coworkers, friends, and even strangers.

Try to focus on everything you have to be thankful for when dealing with a challenging situation. Being grateful for what you have will help you stay positive and will impact everything you do. Also, focus on the things that are within your circle of influence, and don't focus on things outside the circle. This is advice from the book *The Seven Habits of Highly Successful People*. For example, the weather is outside your circle of influence, so don't stress about it, as there's nothing you can do about it.

When your boss has a bad day and takes it out on you, this is also out of your circle of influence.

Try not to waste your time worrying about the things you can't control. Instead, focus on what *is* within your circle of influence, or the things that you can control. One area that this definitely applies to is your fitness and weight-loss journey. At this very moment, you can grab a glass of water, walk for five minutes in your living room, have a healthy snack, or nail your interval workout, and that one step makes you healthier. You are in complete control of being healthier, and I invite you right now to make one decision that moves you in the right direction.

You don't need to sweat how much weight you have to lose or how many workouts you're going to do this week. All you need to do is look at one day at a time and win today! Are you worth it? Yes!

Today, if things go wrong, try to step out of the situation and think about how you can stay positive. Life's too short to sweat the small stuff. We all have a lot to be thankful for (our health and the fact that we can walk, our families, our kids, a house to live in and food to put on the table), so focus today on moving forward and staying positive!

Look, you can re-define the way external events affect your internal dialogue. You can choose to train yourself to react with a positive attitude when things go wrong and develop a new habit of positivity.

There will be few times in your life when the conditions will be better than right now to establish the habit of having a positive attitude because the other elements of this program have positioned you ideally for a radical shift in consciousness. To put it simply, this one habit has the power to transform everything you do from this point on.

ARE YOU WORTH IT? YES!

Are you and your health worth investing your time and energy? Be honest with yourself and please answer this tough question.

Now, do your actions match your answer?

If you answered yes, then you deserve to work this program to meet your fitness and weight-loss goals. If you answered no, then you need to spend some time thinking about why you don't think you are worth investing your time and energy.

Until you realize you are worth it, staying on this program will be challenging because you'll be swimming against the current.

Every one of us deserves to feel good about ourselves, to have tons of energy, and to be healthy. So answer the "are you worth it" question with a loud yes! And then make your actions a reflection of your knowing you are worth it.

Once you do this, your rocket will leave the pad.

YOU DESERVE TO BE HEALTHY AND HAVE TONS OF ENERGY

Once you realize and truly believe that you're worth it, keep reminding yourself why that you deserve to put the time and energy into becoming healthy.

You work hard to keep your house in order, help your kids with their homework, drive them to activities, make meals for your family, and to be a great spouse; you work hard at your job. The list goes on and on, and this leaves you with minimal, if any, personal time. You deserve to have some "me time" each day. By taking time out of your busy schedule to invest in your own health and energy, you will be that much better of a parent, spouse, employee and friend.

What if I told you I could show you a way to manufacture extra time? If fact for every 30 minutes you exercise, you get back hours of energy in return.

Many parents (especially moms) think they cannot or should not take time to exercise most days of the week. But by improving your health and energy and taking time for yourself each day, you will be much better off, and your family and friends will surely benefit.

So today or any day that you're thinking that you can't afford to take time to exercise, instead think about whether you can really afford not to take some me time in order to be the best version of yourself.

You are worth it and deserve to feel healthy and energized!

PROVE TO YOURSELF THAT YOU WERE RIGHT

I read about the following concept in one of my favorite motivational books: *Three Feet from Gold: Turn Your Obstacles into Opportunities!* by Sharon Lechter and Greg Reid.

"Stop trying to prove other people wrong, and focus on proving yourself right!"

Please read the above powerful statement over again a few times.

There's no shortage of doubters in the world:

- You can't do that.
- You won't be able to get fit.
- Is walking your first 5K doable or safe?
- Who are you to walk or run a marathon?
- Didn't you try to lose the weight before?

When friends, family, or anyone else says things like this, they are not necessarily trying to rain on your parade; they're probably just speaking from their own insecurities. It's human nature to try to prove our doubters wrong. But what will happen when you put 100 percent of your focus into proving yourself right?

Your rocket will leave the pad, and you'll shock yourself with who you become.

VISUALIZE THE NEW YOU

I want you to take a few minutes and visualize the new you. Concentrate on how much energy you'll have, how healthy you'll be, and how great you'll look and feel. Imagine you're sitting on a bench and the new, fit, high-energy you comes walking by. What would you see? Just imagine this for a few minutes.

We all remember points in our lives when we were fit, were at a healthy weight, and felt amazing. Maybe it was in high school, before your wedding, or before you had kids. Whenever it was, you can get back to that magical place of feeling like you have unlimited energy. The key is to focus on making healthy decisions one day at a time: win today and repeat!

BELIEVE IN YOURSELF

Believing in yourself and staying positive are so important to reaching your fitness and weight-loss goals. If you don't believe you can do it, then you aren't going to be successful. It is a fact. It's just how it works!

When I told people that I was going to run my first Boston Marathon in 1995 (when I weighed 224 pounds), most of them thought I was crazy. But I believed in myself and took it one day at a time. I went after my dream and made it happen. The same thing happened again five years later when I told people I was going to do my first Ironman Triathlon. Everyone thought I was crazy since I had never taken a swimming lesson and really couldn't swim. But I believed in myself, took it one workout and one day at a time, and achieved that dream.

Eighteen straight Boston Marathons and twelve Ironmans later, I can attest to the power of believing in yourself. This isn't just theory, it works!

You can accomplish all your goals by believing in yourself. The strength necessary to reach the top of any mountain you set your sight on, lies within you. That version of yourself, having unlimited energy and ready to take on anything, is ready to be reintroduced to the world, so believe in yourself and turn your dreams into accomplishments!

DON'T GIVE AWAY YOUR POWER

Just because someone was rude enough to talk you down when you were younger does not mean they have a right to keep robbing you of your happiness. Don't let rude comments from a coach, teacher, parent, or anyone else rob you of today and tomorrow's victories!

When you let hurtful prior experiences hold you back, you are giving away power—power that is yours! Only *your* opinion is the one that truly matters. And only you get to truly judge who you are and, more importantly, who you deserve to be.

I say you decide right now that this is your time to take back the power and to go for it.

I know for a fact that since you're reading this, there's a high-energy, feel-like-a-million-bucks version of you inside of you who is ready to be revealed. Take back your power, and then hit the gas.

CHANGE "WHY CAN'T I" TO "I'M GOING TO"

When we ask ourselves positive and forward-thinking questions, we receive positive and forward-thinking answers. And when we ask ourselves negative and rearview-mirror-thinking questions, we receive negative and rearview-mirror-thinking answers.

Here are a few key examples:

1) Change "Why can't I lose weight?" to "I'm going to lose weight by eating breakfast within one hour of waking up, drinking water all day, exercising, limiting myself to one dessert per week, and getting seven hours of sleep each night."
2) Change "Why can't I fit in my workouts?" to "I'm going to fit in my workouts by refusing to let my negative voice feed me the lie that I don't have time today."
3) Change "Why can't I walk or run my first 5K?" to "I'm going to walk my first 5K by following this program."

When you declare positive and forward-thinking statements instead of asking yourself limited-thinking questions, you immediately start becoming a problem solver and literally start moving in the right direction at that moment. Stop letting your negative voice feed you the garbage that's robbing you of true happiness.

SPEED BUMPS VERSUS ROADBLOCKS

Many people fall off of their exercise routine or healthy eating habits and then give up. They view one bad day or a bad week as a roadblock. But you should look at setbacks as speed bumps—not roadblocks.

So you had a bad day or week; that's no reason to beat yourself up or give up. Today is a new day! At any given time, you are one decision away from making today a great day and getting back on track.

Remember, you can't change yesterday. Beating yourself up over missed workouts or overeating will not do you any good. So forget about turning bad days into roadblocks and instead look at them as speed bumps. They slow you down a little, but hit the gas, and you'll be right back on your way.

BEING ABLE TO WALK IS A TRUE GIFT

It's easy to rush through life and overlook how much you have to be thankful for. When you're feeling tired or down for any reason, it's easy to forget that there are untold numbers of people in this world who would do anything to be able to walk, much less do a workout. Being able to walk is a true gift!

Patrick Henry Hughes is blind and in a wheelchair, and his "attitude of gratitude" and positive thinking are truly remarkable. Go to www.NoExcusesWorkouts.com/Book to view a quick and powerful video about Patrick. Get ready to shed tears of joy. This video is as powerful as they come.

Embrace how lucky you are to be able to walk, run and smile—you are truly blessed. Being grateful for your gifts will have a significant impact on your attitude and life. Think about this the next time you're having trouble starting a workout. While you're exercising, smile and be thankful for the gift of good health!

BE GRATEFUL

You deserve to have a stress-free fitness and weight-loss journey. Life's too short to worry all the time and to be lectured by your negative voice about your weight and how you gained it.

I want you to commit right now to spending three full days focusing on everything you have to be grateful for: your health, your family, having a roof over your head and having food in the fridge.

The truth is, there are many people in this world who are really banged up and would give their right arm to be in your shoes. Yes, we all have our struggles. But if your biggest struggle is losing weight, then as your coach let me just say that you're fine and it's all going to come together.

Focus on being grateful for all you have to be thankful for, follow my lead, and enjoy your stress-free ride to becoming the high-energy version of yourself that you deserve to be.

A FOCUSED MISSION

Spend five minutes with no TV, radio, or distractions thinking about everything you have to be grateful for. Then, write a list of the ten things you are most grateful for. Carry this list around with you all day, and reread it every hour.

When you shift into a spot of being truly grateful for everything you have, you're in a mentally strong position to make your health a top priority and to take action. Being grateful changes everything!

THERE'S NO HOT WATER TODAY

One day, the person at the front desk of my gym told me that there was no hot water. I then said, "At least there's water," and he smiled. A lot of people at the desk were upset about the "huge" cold-shower problem.

While I was working out, I was thinking about having to take a freezing-cold shower. I thought, "There are between one and two billion people in this world with no running water, so I can handle this today."

How do you react when things that are out of your control go wrong? The answer to this question says a lot about whether you will be successful in reaching your fitness and weight-loss goals. Let me support you in finding ways to turn less than ideal situations into opportunities for growth in your life. Go to http://www.NoExcusesWorkouts.com/ and lets all start looking at the glass as half-full, and learn to roll with the punches.

By the way, remember that cold shower I was getting ready for? Well, the showers were fixed before I finished my workout, and I felt like I'd been rewarded with a warm shower for staying positive. How would you react if the person at your gym told you there was no hot water today?

THE LAW OF ATTRACTION

Have you read *The Secret*? If so, you know the central theme is the law of attraction. If you haven't read it, I suggest you pick up a copy.

You don't have to buy into all the concepts, but I do want you to think about the law of attraction, which says that you will attract people and things to you based on the energy you give out and based on what you think about.

If you're a positive person, you will attract positive people and positive things. If you're a negative person, you will attract negative people and negative things.

Are you a generally positive person? Do you have positive friends and a generally positive family?

None of us are perfect. But today, I want you to really think about staying positive and attracting positive people and positive things into your world.

Also, if you have people in your world who are draining your energy, think about what you can do to change their negativity. Or make the very difficult decision to spend less time with the people who are dragging you in the wrong direction. One way or another, protect your energy.

Having a positive outlook has a great impact on everything from how you respond to problems to how successful you are in losing weight and getting fit, to how much you enjoy your job, to how much fun you have with your family.

From this day on, focus on staying positive and the law of attraction will be working for you!

CHAPTER 11: CELEBRATE SMALL WINS

YOU'RE STRONGER THAN YOU REALIZE

Most of us (me included) are only using a fraction of the amazing gifts we have been given. Think about it for a second—it's true. You and I don't even realize how many gifts we possess and how much untapped potential lies within us.

Please read through the following powerful quote at least three times and then take three to five minutes to realize how strong you are. Think about what you've been afraid of doing, and realize that you definitely have the strength to accomplish your goals.

"Deep within man dwell those slumbering powers; powers that would astonish him, that he never dreamed of possessing; forces that would revolutionize his life if aroused and put into action."
— Orison Swett Marden

GO AT YOUR OWN PACE

When it comes to working out, forget about what everyone else is doing and concentrate on what *you* are doing. If you go to a gym, don't worry about the person next to you who's sweating like crazy and has been on her treadmill for sixty minutes. Instead, focus on taking small and healthy steps toward improving your health.

If you're new to exercise, than you should err on the side of caution and take it slow out of the gate. Remember, you don't want to sprint at the beginning of a marathon!

When you do the No Excuses Workout, don't worry if you can only do one or two push-ups against the wall when you first start. One is ten times more than zero, and the less you can do initially, the more excited you should be about the progress you are going to make.

When you do Interval Workouts, start off by doing ten minutes, and know that just ten minutes is a beautiful thing: Every time you move it helps improve your health! Focus all of your energy on doing safe and effective workouts that are right for you, and literally forget about everyone else.

I'm not encouraging you to slack off, I am urging you to take it at your own pace. By doing that, you'll avoid injury and burnout, and you'll set yourself up to create true lifestyle changes. Stay safe and have fun!

FOCUS ON BEING IN THE GAME

We all have struggles on our fitness and weight-loss journeys. When struggles arise, it's so easy to forget the big picture and instead obsess about what's going wrong in the moment and how easy it would be to just quit. I feel this way at times, although I try my best to push through these feelings, knowing that in the long run, I will feel better for it.

To be successful in your efforts to get in amazing shape and lose weight, you must be "in the game."

"In the game" means you do three push-ups against the wall rather than blowing off your No Excuses workout because you can't do a push-up from your knees yet.

"In the game" means doing a five-minute walk around your neighborhood if you're just getting started, and being proud of it.

"In the game" is not judging yourself about whether you're running seventeen-minute miles or eight-minute miles.

"In the game" is doing a twelve-minute interval workout instead of missing the whole workout because you can't do the full 30 minutes.

Forget your pace. Forget your amount of workout time. Be "in the game" and celebrate it. No excuses!

STOP AND BE PROUD

If you've been staying consistent with your workouts, then stop and reflect on what you've been doing and what you've accomplished! Many times we're rushing through life and forget to slow down, take an assessment and then be proud of ourselves for our accomplishments.

Taking the stairs instead of the elevator, parking in the farthest spot at the grocery store, drinking sixty-four ounces of water during the day, and doing your interval or No Excuses Workouts, should all be celebrated.

Take the time to be proud of yourself, and don't minimalize the small changes that you're making to improve your health. By celebrating your small victories, you'll have a heightened sense of accomplishment that will definitely keep feeding your motivation and results. The small victories lead to more small victories, which lead to more energy, weight loss, and health improvements. You will feel amazing, and that's what you deserve!

So regardless of how small the step, celebrate your small victories! Smile and be proud! You're doing it, and you're setting yourself up to be the healthiest version of yourself possible.

Take five or ten minutes to think about what you've accomplished. It doesn't matter if you haven't lost a pound yet—if you're staying consistent with your workouts and making healthy food choices, then you are probably doing all four of these amazing things:

1) Increasing your energy
2) Improving your mood
3) Improving your health and self-image
4) Serving as an example of health to your kids and family

If you've been having trouble staying motivated and have let your workouts slip, it's not too late. Jump in today and make a few healthy choices. Beating yourself up over yesterday isn't going to help you. Today is a fresh start, and by jumping back in you'll be back cranking before you know it!

IS GOOD ENOUGH REALLY GOOD ENOUGH?

The saying "good enough" can be taken two ways.

If you use "good enough" to describe your decision to blow off your last interval within your interval workout then it really is not "good enough."

If you use "good enough" to describe the fact that you didn't do your formal interval workout yesterday because the kids were sick but you still fit in some random acts of fitness around the house, then it really is "good enough."

There is a difference between achieving small victories and cheating. Cheating is not OK. Only you know if "good enough" is really "good enough". Stop saying "good enough" if it really isn't. And start saying "good enough" if it really is.

REWARD YOURSELF

Have you been rewarding yourself for staying consistent with your exercise and losing weight? If not, I suggest you consider setting up rewards for accomplishing your fitness and weight-loss goals.

Here are some reasons for rewarding yourself:

- You've averaged three Interval Workouts and three No Excuses Workouts per week for three weeks.
- You've lost five pounds.
- You've only had dessert once per week for three weeks.
- You've not skipped a meal in three weeks.
- You've been sweating every time you do an interval workout for the last three weeks.
- You've been drinking sixty-four ounces of water per day for three weeks.

Set up specific goals, and then pick a fun reward for your accomplishments. Here are some examples of potential rewards:

- a new water bottle
- a massage
- a new pair of sneakers
- new workout clothes
- a manicure
- a nice lunch or dinner with your spouse, partner, or best friend
- a book you've been wanting to order for a while

By setting up fun rewards for your hard work, you add additional incentive to stay consistent and reach your goals. So pick something fun and get after it!

CELEBRATE WHO YOU ARE INSTEAD OF DWELLING ON WHO YOU AREN'T

What would happen if you focused on being proud of who you are and what you do (a great parent, staying active, trying your best and so on) instead of dwelling on what you don't do?

The negative voice in your head is constantly trying to talk you down because of missed opportunities, missed workouts, and weight gained. But the positive voice in your head is trying to get you to see how well you're doing. Being a wonderful parent and a good person is one hundred times more important than fitting in skinny jeans, isn't it? Your positive voice wants you to celebrate your small wins and to focus on all the great things you're doing for your body and mind. And I want you to get real!

Be proud and celebrate who you are and focus on listening to the positive voice in your head!

CHAPTER 12: SURROUND YOURSELF WITH POSITIVE PEOPLE

"Most people are a direct reflection of the aspirations of their five closest friends."
— Tony Robbins

MINIMIZE YOUR EXPOSURE TO NEGATIVE PEOPLE

How many negative people do you have in your life? Do you have negative friends or family members who drag you down? Negative people suck the energy out of all of us. They talk about how tough everything is, how unhappy they are, and how difficult life is—and most of the time they drag us down with them.

We all have bad days, but you need to be careful about spending too much time with negative people who take you in the wrong direction. I'm very guarded about letting people drag me down, and you should be as well.

Let's look at an example. On a scale of one to five where five is extremely positive and one is extremely negative, if you and I get together and you are a five and I am a one, then by the end of our talk we are both threes. You lifted me up, and I dragged you down.

As you start to take on new, healthy habits you may feel that some people in your world are trying to drag you in the wrong direction.

This isn't because they don't care about you, it's because your healthy choices can make them feel uncomfortable. As spectators, the fact that they are not achieving their potential becomes painfully evident as they watch your rocket leave the pad. It's critical that you communicate how important your new, healthy habits are to your friends, family, and coworkers. Having a few simple conversations about how you need your support network to stay positive and encourage you. You will protect your progress by being vocal about your needs.

Unfortunately sometimes you are going to need to make the tough decision that certain friends are only going to drag you down, be negative, and not embrace the new you. This is tough, but it's sometimes best to move on. I'm not telling you to ditch your friends, but I am asking you to be guarded about allowing people to stop you from becoming who you deserve to be.

I want to illustrate this key concept with a story:

Back in the late nineties, after I had lost forty pounds and had run a few Boston Marathons, my "friends" would continually harass me about being "Mr. Fitness" or "Mr. Energy". They meant well, but after trying to deflect their comments and eventually even having the tough "if you're not going to say anything positive don't say anything at all" conversations, they kept at it. Finally, I hit my breaking point.

We had all rented a house on Nantucket for a week, and the first night my friends partied, got drunk, and as usual were self-destructive. In the morning I got up early and went for a ten-mile run along on the water. I felt amazing, and I was on fire when I got back to the house. My "friends" were all hungover, and they literally could not let it go that "Mr. Fitness" had run ten miles while they were all sleeping. It went on all day and night. That night I hit my breaking point; I left the bar early, went home, and went to bed. The next morning, I got up, packed my bags, told my soon-to-be-former "friends" that I'd had enough and I was leaving. I got a cab, hopped on a ferry, and on day three of our week-long (and expensive) vacation, I was out of there.

That decision proved to be one of the best decisions of my life because over the next one to three years I went through a significant friend upgrade from deadweights to winners. And not surprisingly, my own life (both personally and professionally) soared! Is it time for you to upgrade your friends too?

DON'T LISTEN TO THE DOUBTERS

If we listen to the family members, friends, neighbors and coworkers who doubt us, then we will never accomplish anything!

As we discussed earlier, many times these people are not trying to discourage us but are dealing with their own insecurities. So when you talk about walking your first 5K or losing forty pounds, people sometimes get uncomfortable and react by trying to talk you out of chasing down your goals.

If I'd listened to the doubters when I weighed 224 pounds and was wearing size thirty-eight pants and decided not to run my first Boston Marathon back in 1995, I would not be who I am or where I am today. No matter what anyone around you thinks or says, you can accomplish anything you set your mind to. You just need to take it one step at a time, stay consistent with your workouts, and keep it fun.

NEGATIVE COMMENTS FROM FAMILY MEMBERS

Getting together with family or friends during the holidays or other events is usually fun.

But when your mom, aunt, sister or friend start making negative comments about the weight you have lost, it can turn a fun time into an uncomfortable one very quickly.

When people see others thriving (especially successfully losing weight), they start asking themselves tough questions like "How come I'm not doing that?" and this leads to feelings of insecurity and generates negative comments. The best advice I can give you is to kill them with your kindness with replies like "I'm actually doing this the healthy way by exercising and eating right. And the great thing is, I'm having fun and I feel amazing."

If killing them with your kindness doesn't work, you may have to resort to a firmer response such as "To be honest, if you don't have anything nice to say about my weight loss, then please don't comment on it." You've worked too hard and come too far to let anyone rain on your parade.

BECOME A POSITIVE CONTENT MACHINE

"Stand guard at the gates to your mind!"
— Jim Rohn

We're focusing on the importance of surrounding ourselves with positive winners in this section because we match the speed of our peers. In addition to suggesting that you surround yourself with positive people, I suggest you look at what you're watching, what you're listening to, and what you're reading for additional opportunities to crank up your positivity, energy, mood, weight loss, fitness, health, and life!

- What do you watch?
- What do you listen to?
- What do you read?

Grab a piece of paper and write down your answers to the above three questions, and then mark each answer with a P for positive or an N for negative.

Each time we consume content (watch it, listen to it, or read it), we are either lifting ourselves up or dragging ourselves down. And if you spend any time in the car then you have a tremendous opportunity to use that time to consumer positive content.

"Turn your car into a mobile classroom."
— Zig Ziglar

Here's something fun to consider: your fitness and weight-loss results (and probably your entire life) will take off when you swap many of your negative sources of content for positive ones. Give it a try for one week, and see what this does for your energy and mood along with your fitness and weight-loss goals! Remember, garbage in equals garbage out and positivity in equals positivity out!

CHAPTER 13: HABITS LEAD TO RESULTS

In the Introduction I shared my Fifteen Secrets to Better Health. As I mentioned there, those 15 habits are your roadmap to the results you deserve. And as you are about to read, it is our habits that lead to lasting results.

REMOVE THE GRAY AREA

You deserve to be losing one to three pounds per week and to feel amazing. Removing any gray area from what you're doing is one of the keys to getting there. Let me explain: you have to take your "winging it" hat off and add definition to what you're doing. Saying, "I'm going to exercise on Friday" is too gray. Make it black and white. Add definition and accountability to what you're doing by writing your workout in your calendar for a set time, such as Friday at 9AM.

Winging it doesn't work because we get busier and busier as the day goes on, and "later today" becomes "OK, I'll have to take care of it tomorrow" and tomorrow never comes. The busier you are (especially if you're a mom), the more you need to pick the days and times to exercise and write them in your calendar. By planning this out in advance, you will set yourself up to stay consistent and be successful in reaching your fitness and weight-loss goals.

Since you're now committed to accomplishing your goals, you deserve to have a set plan. To stay consistent with your workouts and to achieve results, you need to commit to specific days and times. You also need to write these in your calendar as appointments with yourself that you really cannot miss. You wouldn't skip a meeting for work or for your child at school, so how can you skip a workout meeting with yourself? This is another great way to focus on making your health a priority.

WIN TODAY AND TOMORROW

The best way to win tomorrow is to prepare for tomorrow's success tonight. And the best way to win today is to keep track of your healthy decisions all throughout the day.

Use the Win Tomorrow and Win Today checklists, which you can download at www.NoExcusesWorkouts.com/Book, so that you can set yourself up to be successful tomorrow and then track your success during the day.

Why the Win Tomorrow checklist is so important:

- With a busy schedule, it is really important to set yourself up to win each day by taking action the night before.
- By having these key things ready in advance you remove the possibility of results-robbing excuses.

Why the Win Today checklist is so important:

- Winging it doesn't work, so this list provides you with a game-plan to follow each day.

If you score a consistent 35 or more on your Win Tomorrow and Win Today scores, you should lose an average of one to three pounds per week and crank up your fitness results!

There are 1,440 minutes per day, so you can easily afford ten minutes to complete these important checklists. Go to www.NoExcusesWorkouts.com/Book to print out the checklists. Do it now! It's time to get started.

THE WIN TOMORROW CHECKLIST

Use this checklist to get you ready to make healthy food choices and nail your workout tomorrow.

	Completed? (Enter 0 or 1)						
ACTION ITEM	Mon.	Tue.	Wed.	Thu.	Fri.	Sat.	Sun.
Get your water bottles ready.							
Get your healthy snacks ready.							
Make or plan your lunch.							
Get your workout clothes and sneakers ready.							
Schedule tomorrow's work-out in your calendar.							
Set an exact bedtime for tonight.							
TOTAL SCORE							
WIN TOMORROW SCORE FOR THE WEEK (MAX = 42):							

THE WIN TODAY CHECKLIST

Use this checklist to keep you on track each day.

	Completed? (Enter 0 or 1)						
ACTION ITEM	Mon.	Tue.	Wed.	Thu.	Fri.	Sat.	Sun.
Had breakfast within 1 hour of waking							
Had a healthy mid-morning snack							
Drank plenty of water (all day long)							
Nailed my scheduled workout							
Did Random Acts of Fitness throughout the day							
Had a healthy mid-afternoon snack							
Controlled my portions at lunch and dinner							
Only had dessert if this was my one dessert night							
Went to bed at a set time to line me up for seven hours							
TOTAL SCORE							

10 OUT OF 1,440 MINUTES

The people who accomplish amazing things in life (including hitting their goal weight and getting fit and staying there) make the important decision to allocate a certain amount of time to their health.

Be accountable! As I had you do earlier, it's time to add up the hours you spend each day online and watching TV. I want you to access how easily you can fit in these important ten planning minutes.

If you commit to these ten minutes out of your available 1,440 minutes each day, you'll be shocked how much this one habit will crank up your fitness and weight-loss results!

IMPROVE YOUR HEALTH ONE BRICK AT A TIME

I want you to think of improving your health in terms of building a house. Each day you're trying to add a few bricks to the house. The more healthy decisions you make, the more bricks you add each day. Some days when you feel great and are making many healthy choices, you add ten bricks to the house. Some days when you're struggling, you still manage to add a few bricks to the house. And some days you may not be able to add any bricks at all.

You can't build a house in a day or a week, and you can't achieve optimal health that quickly either. To build a quality house that will last takes time. And losing weight, keeping it off, and improving your health takes time. So today and as you move forward, think of improving your health as building a house. Do it one brick at a time by taking small steps and making smart choices. Before you know it you'll have a solid foundation and ultimately you will build a house that will last.

FOCUS ON THE PROCESS, NOT RESULTS

We're all wired to focus on results: How much weight have you lost? How many inches have you lost? How much has your energy gone up? Blah, blah, blah! Sound familiar? Yes, results are fantastic, and there's no better feeling than being fit and having tons of energy. **But the path to that place is paved by your habits.**

Form healthy habits: drink plenty of water, park far from the door, have dessert once per week, nail your workouts and stay positive and the results will follow. I invite you to take it one day at a time. Focus on building healthy habits and forget about achieving exact results.

This will be a less stressful journey and ultimately lead you to the success you deserve.

PICK A FEW EASY WINS

Most people shoot for drastic changes when they attempt to lose weight. They decide "now is the time" and jump in with both feet. This is how most people are at the beginning of January during New Years' resolution time. But the problem with this approach is that it rarely works. This is because completely cutting yourself off from certain foods or trying to take an hour out of each day to exercise isn't sustainable.

As soon as our new habits start infringing too much on our current lifestyles or it starts feeling like a part-time job, we bail. Not because we're slackers or are abnormal. It's just because we're human, and when we shoot for drastic change, it rarely plays out.

Here is a simple approach that truly works: pick a few easy wins, and then nail them!

Once those few habits stick you can then choose one to two more healthy habits to focus on. Please refer to the 15 Secrets to Better Health to select your next one or two key habits.

Once you nail your easy wins for a few weeks, you'll prove to yourself that you can build and sustain healthy habits. Then it's simply a process of repeating the same approach and continuing to layer on new healthy habits. This is the process to use to achieve sustained optimal health and permanent weight loss.

WIN TODAY AND REPEAT

You deserve to look at your workouts and weight-loss journey as a source of power and not as something that adds stress to your life. It's easy to get stressed or psyched out by the thought of having to lose a certain number of pounds, work out five to six days per week, or eat dessert only once per week.

I invite you instead to keep things simple: focus on one day a time and one healthy decision at a time.

Then win today and repeat! When you do that, your daily victories start to link together, and before you know it you feel great, have tons of energy, and have lost weight. By simplifying your weight-loss journey down to one decision and one day at a time, you free yourself to build healthy habits. And when you build the right habits, the fitness and weight-loss results always follow.

Free yourself from the stress of trying to chase down specific weight-loss goals and instead put 100 percent of your effort into the process. When you focus on one day at a time and one healthy decision at a time, you are able to build lasting habits.

IS SPENDING TOO MUCH TIME ONLINE HURTING YOUR HEALTH?

Are you spending so much time online (e-mails, forums, Twitter and Facebook) that you aren't fitting in your workouts? If so, I suggest you limit yourself to thirty minutes of Internet time each day unless you've done your workout. This will be hard at first, but it will shock you how much holding yourself accountable to this rule will improve your workout consistency and results. Your health is too important to overlook, so please follow my lead on this and control your time online!

If you need convincing, please complete the following exercise:

1) Add up the average amount of time you spend watching TV and online each day.
2) Add up the average amount of time you spend exercising each day.

Listen, just think what would happen if you took thirty minutes from number one (your TV and online time) and flipped it to number two (your exercise time). Your life would change forever! You would probably hit your goal weight and more importantly have unlimited energy and feel truly amazing! Seriously, what is it going to cost you? A TV Show? A Facebook Post? Aren't you willing to make this one simple change in order to transform your life forever?

BEER VERSUS TOMATO JUICE

I once sat next to two contrasting health examples on a flight: A guy who was around forty and was about fifty pounds overweight, and a guy who was around sixty and seemed to be at a great weight, was healthy, and had tons of positive energy.

When it came time to order a drink, the first guy ordered a beer and the second guy ordered a tomato juice. Guy number one had nothing else to drink for the next two hours and guy number two was drinking out of a big water bottle. To me, their drink orders spoke volumes about how they each prioritized their health.

I wanted to talk with the guy with the beer so that I could see if he would be interested in joining the free No Excuses Team or trying out our free workouts. But when he was rude to the young girl in front of us, I decided that talking with him would be a waste of time. The truth is, we create our lives one good or one bad decision at a time.

Yes, you are what you eat and drink! What you eat on a regular basis (fruits and veggies versus junk food, a healthy salad versus a bacon cheeseburger with fries, tomato juice versus beer) is just as important as investing time to work out most days of the week. As you can see, making healthy daily food choices is a major investment in your health and your outlook.

EVERYTHING IN MODERATION

Taking an all-or-nothing approach to your eating can be as unproductive as taking that same approach to your exercise.

When you try to completely cut yourself off from the things you love, you inevitably finally give up. Does this sound like what happens when you diet? You restrict yourself from something you love, and then when you can't take it anymore, you inhale large quantities of it. It really is torture to avoid foods you like even when you know they're unhealthy for you. When you make a certain food "forbidden," what you're really doing is giving that food more power than it deserves. It can stir up a great deal of emotions and make you focus more on what you can't have than on what you can. As the saying goes, what you resist persists.

I invite you to always keep in mind the term "everything in moderation". It's not going to kill you to occasionally have a cheeseburger, a few beers or a bowl of ice cream. The problem is when you let yourself get overly hungry and then feel the need to eat a large quantity of something that isn't healthy for you. Instead of putting your energy into avoiding a certain food, try to manage your hunger so that you're never desperate, This way you can fill up on healthy foods a majority of the time and allow yourself a treat every now and then. This is the strategy behind having dessert one night per week! I want you to get healthy and I want you to enjoy the things that you like to, and that includes your favorite dessert.

SET WEEKLY MINIMUMS

Success with healthy lifestyle changes also comes from creating exercise habits. One way to do this is to set a certain amount of movement that you're going to do each week no matter what; What I mean is that you should make a commitment to, for example, three 15-minute Interval Workouts and three six-minute No Excuses Workouts per week - no excuses! In this example you're committing to yourself to do at least 63 minutes of exercise per week. This would be your "lower limit," or the minimum amount of exercise you will complete each week. If you can do more, great! But even if you have a challenging week, you've made a commitment to yourself that you'll fit in a certain amount of movement.

Setting this lower limit is important both physically and mentally. If you stick to your minimum you'll never really fall out of shape, and you won't beat yourself up for letting a week go by where you didn't do at least some positive movement.

THE IMPORTANCE OF TRACKING YOUR WORKOUTS

Another great way to increase fitness habits is to track your workouts. Are you tracking your workouts? If not, I suggest you start doing so as an additional source of motivation and accountability. By having a record of your hard work, you're able to look back on what you did right on the weeks when you're happy with your results and what you may or may not have done on other weeks when you're disappointed.

You should start seeing this trend and feel very motivated: The weeks you're consistent with doing three

Interval Workouts and three No Excuses Workouts are the weeks when you are happy with your results and feel great!

Again, this is a great way to stay motivated and accountable to yourself.

RANDOM ACTS OF FITNESS

Yet another way to create healthy habits and increase your overall daily movement is to fit in Random Acts of Fitness. You will be amazed how much exercise you can fit in without even putting on workout clothes. You can also put on your creative hat and have fun thinking up ways that you and your entire family can add in Random Acts of Fitness.

Here are a few examples:

1) March in place while brushing your teeth in the morning and evening (twice a day for two to three minutes equals four to six minutes of exercise).
2) Take an extra trip to the mailbox and back when you grab your mail (you may look strange to your neighbors, but who cares if it helps you feel like a million bucks).
3) Take the stairs at work, the mall, or whenever you normally would take an elevator.

4) Park in the farthest spot in the lot at your office, grocery store or mall.
5) Walk up and down your stairs (or march in place) during the commercials while watching TV. The average one-hour show has seventeen minutes of commercials, so moving during commercials is a great way to improve your health and stay active.

I also suggest you turn some of your cleaning routines around the house into Random Acts of Fitness. All you need to do is be creative about what things you can do to get your heart rate up and work your muscles.

To help you get going, I want you to make your own list of at least five ways you can add Random Acts of Fitness to your life. Once you start adding these into your routine, they'll become habit, and you'll be amazed by the effect it can have. This extra daily movement is not only good for you but also sends a positive signal to yourself that your health is important and is a top priority.

WHY WOULD YOU WALK?

One Random Act of Fitness that I always try to do is to walk whenever I can. For example, when Karen, Alexander, Benjamin, and I travel, we walk from one terminal to the other any time we have a connecting flight.

This is a great way to fit in additional movement, and we make this a fun time for all of us!

During one of our trips, when we asked one of the airport employees for directions to our terminal, he pointed us to the shuttle. We explained that we wanted to walk and he said, "Just take the shuttle - it's easier, and it's too far to walk." We insisted that we wanted to walk to which he replied: "Take a right out the door and just keep walking."

He added, "Why would you walk when you can take the shuttle?" It was a sad statement and says a lot about why our country is in the middle of an obesity epidemic.

While we were walking, one of the shuttles pulled over and opened the door (which was very nice since the driver saw us with our children and also pulling our luggage). I said, "Thanks, but we are all set—we're walking." The driver looked at me like I had two heads.

To be healthy and have tons of energy, you have to sometimes avoid the easy way out. At the airport, shopping mall, or the office, I still park the car in the far corner of the parking lot, and I always take the stairs. I do this because I love practicing what I preach and because I want to keep these healthy habits going.

Did you take the stairs today? Did you park in one of the farthest spots at the office or grocery store? These small choices will add up to have a significant positive impact on your energy and health. Make the healthy choice for you and for your family.

CHAPTER 14: QUICK WORKOUTS ARE THE KEY TO SUCCESS

EXERCISE SHOULDN'T BE A PART-TIME JOB

Spending big chunks of time exercising is zero fun and ends up robbing you of time you could spend playing with your kids, reading a book, relaxing, or doing something else you love. When the quality of your workouts is high and you're maximizing your results by doing intervals and No Excuses Workouts, you don't have to exercise for more than thirty minutes per day.

Are you doing quality workouts, or are you just going through the motions and "putting in your time"? If you're exercising for more than thirty minutes per day and aren't happy with your results, then please change your approach and focus on the quality of your workouts.

Doing quality workouts enables you to avoid feeling like exercising is a part-time job and keeps it fun.

You maximize your results in quick windows of time and know that every minute invested is a step in the right direction to crank up your energy and improve your health.

Jump on the Interval Workout and No Excuses Workout train, and you'll feel like a rock star by exercising an efficient thirty minutes per day!

ENERGY UP, MOOD UP

Instead of looking at exercise as a way to lose weight and get healthy, focus on using it purely to crank up your energy and mood. When you do that, it moves up your priority list, and you start using exercise as your number-one tool to feel amazing and to be your best you.

The person you are when you finish a workout is always a more positive, upbeat, and happy version of yourself. And everyone who spends time around you wins!

When you focus on using your workouts solely to crank up your energy and mood, you remove the stress related to "I have to exercise to lose weight," and the weight loss takes care of itself.

NO PAIN, NO GAIN ISN'T TRUE

There's a common saying in fitness: no pain, no gain. But this is definitely not true.

You should never be in pain during or after working out. Yes, you should sweat and test yourself, and you should be aware later in the day and the next day that you exercised. But working out to a level where you're in pain increases your risk of injury and burnout and will probably leave you feeling demoralized. Plus, hammering yourself is zero fun and will increase the likelihood of your ditching your workout routine.

Instead of saying No Pain, No Gain, try this affirmation to encourage yourself along the way: No sweat, I am not there yet!

Unless you're within two weeks of starting to exercise or your doctor has instructed you to take it easy, then you really should be sweating during your workouts in order to maximize your results. Sweating is the sign that you're working hard (not to a level of pain, but a solid effort) and helps you maximize your calorie burning and overall results.

So when you're doing your workouts, push yourself so that you're sweating, and be proud!

JUST FIFTEEN MINUTES

In a study of 416,000 people over a thirteen-year period, researchers found that doing just fifteen minutes of moderate exercise a day may add three years to your life. There is now solid research to support the notion that every step counts, and doing even fifteen minutes of exercise daily is beneficial from a health standpoint.

To read the full article about this amazing research, go to www.NoExcusesWorkouts.com/Book

Here's something amazing to consider: If exercising for fifteen minutes per day can add three years to your life, what can thirty minutes do?

WHAT IS A WORKOUT?

A lot of people think they've only done a workout if they do at least thirty minutes and sweat. That's not true! Part of the reason I've been able to keep forty pounds off for eighteen years is because I have redefined the term workout.

I consider a workout to be anything that gets your heart rate up or works your muscles more than sitting in a chair. Here are a few examples:

- Gardening
- Doing laundry by putting only one or two pieces of clothing away at a time
- Cleaning the windows in your house
- Walking to the mailbox and back
- Marching in place while you brush your teeth
- Sweeping your garage

I often do a four-minute workout in my kitchen at night by marching in place while filling up my water bottles and making my lunch for the next day. Strange—yes. But also effective! As you can see from my examples, you can turn some of your house projects and routines into workouts and create a true win-win scenario. So be creative, and you'll be pleasantly surprised how active you are and how consistent you are with your workouts.

Yes, I still suggest you nail three Interval Workouts and three No Excuses Workouts per week. But doing a bunch of other random workouts will help crank up your results.

As you now know, you don't have to be at a gym or sweating to fit in extra workouts during the day. All you need to do is either get your heart rate up or work your muscles a little more than usual, and you're definitely doing a workout.

THE MYTH OF THE FAT-BURNING ZONE

When it comes to weight loss, it's all about the total calories burned, not the type of calories burned. So exercising in your fat-burning zone isn't the best way to lose weight or keep it off.

Let me explain with the following two workout examples:

> Workout #1: Exercise for thirty minutes in your fat-burning zone, and burn 300 total calories including 50 percent of your calories as fat and 50 percent as carbohydrates. This is called the fat-burning zone because you're burning more fat as a percentage of calories burned.

> Workout #2: Exercise for thirty minutes doing an Interval Workout or something else that is higher intensity, and burn 450 calories including 33 percent from fat (or 150 calories) and 67 percent from carbohydrates (or 300 calories).

In the second workout, you burn just as many fat calories, but you burn an additional 150 carbohydrate calories. So if you're exercising six days per week, you will burn an additional 900 calories per week. And since a 3,500-calorie difference (between burned and consumed) leads to approximately one pound of weight loss, you would lose an additional thirteen pounds per year. This example doesn't even take into consideration that your metabolism stays elevated for up to twelve hours after each interval workout and the additional contribution this makes to your weight loss.

The point is, whether you burn fat or carbohydrates is not the key factor for weight loss! The key is total calories burned. So get out there and sweat, do your Interval Workouts three times per week, and be proud of yourself for maximizing your fitness and weight-loss results.

BORING WORKOUTS LEAD TO NO WORKOUTS

If your workouts are boring, then the chances of your sticking with them long term is almost zero. The key to staying consistent with your workouts is to find things you love or enjoy doing. Mixing up your workouts is also key.

Think of the sports you enjoyed when you were younger, and consider jumping back in. I started playing basketball again after a seven-year break, and I love it. Even though I'm not very good, I have a blast and get an amazing workout.

Find fun activities or workouts, and your chances of exercising consistently for the long-haul will go up considerably. Remember, fun is easy!

INTERVALS CRANK UP YOUR RESULTS

Since you want to get as fit as possible and lose the most weight you can, you're crazy if you're not doing three Interval Workouts per week!

Intervals not only help you burn 30 percent more calories per workout (versus exercising at a set pace) but they also leave your metabolism elevated for up to twelve hours after each workout. Take it from me, there's nothing better you can do than Interval Training.

Here's an explanation of what makes intervals so effective: most people do steady-state exercise, which means they work up to a level and then stay there for an extended period of time. Of course, this is better than not working out at all, but it isn't the most effective way to maximize your results.

During Interval Training, you'll increase and decrease your exertion levels several times during your routine. You will strive for progressively higher levels of perceived exertion or heart rate for several minutes at a time. In between these push periods you will have one or two minute periods of recovery. For example, the push could involve a quick-paced walk and the recovery could be a slow walk. By pushing your effort level up and down, this taxes your body and causes it to work harder and burn more calories than exercising at one set level. Also, by adding the rest periods in between, you're able to exercise at a higher level during the push intervals and therefore burn that many more calories than staying at one set pace.

Intervals are not only the best way to lose weight; they are also the best way to strengthen your heart and lungs and improve your recovery rates. To get more toned and to perform your best either walking or running your next 5K, 10K, half marathon, or marathon, use Interval Workouts as your secret weapon.

Trust me, I lost 40 pounds eighteen years ago and have kept it off doing Intervals. Plus Intervals are at the core of why I've been able to start and finish twelve Ironman Triathlons and eighteen straight Boston Marathons without hammering my body or feeling like my training is a part-time job.

The great thing about Interval Workouts is that you can do them anywhere (in your living room, outside or at a gym) and when doing any activity you want—all that matters is that you hit the target levels.

You deserve to burn 30 percent more calories per workout and to leave your post-workout metabolism elevated for up to twelve hours. So get after it and make sure to crush your Interval Workouts!

THE #1 WAY TO GET RID OF BELLY FAT

I often get asked what is the best way to reduce excess weight around your core. The answer is to do

Interval Workouts. Although keeping active and doing any movement is great for your health, you need to commit to doing three Interval Workouts per week in order to crank up your metabolism and to trim down your core (and your whole body).

Intervals are definitely the best way to reduce body fat, particularly in your core. Let me emphasize clearly, there is no such thing as spot reduction. You should definitely be doing core work to firm up the muscles in your stomach and lower back, but that won't trim down your core. However, combining core work with Interval Workouts is a powerful one-two punch. The Intervals will help you lose weight, and the core work will help you build muscle and make your core stronger.

INTERVAL WORKOUTS IN THE PRESS

The power of Interval Training has been receiving a lot of positive press. Here are the excerpts from the following three articles:

ARTICLE #1: MAYO CLINIC: REV UP YOUR WORKOUT WITH INTERVAL TRAINING

"Once the domain of elite athletes, interval training has become a powerful tool for the average exerciser, too."

"It's not as complicated as you might think. Interval training is simply alternating bursts of intense activity with intervals of lighter activity."

"You'll burn more calories. The more vigorously you exercise, the more calories you'll burn—even if you increase intensity for just a few minutes at a time."

To read the full article go to www.NoExcuses Workouts.com/Book

ARTICLE #2: CONSUMER REPORTS: INTERVAL TRAINING: MORE BENEFIT, LESS FATIGUE

"The interval method—applicable to virtually any aerobic activity and an option on most exercise machines—avoids long periods of strenuous exercise."

> "That 30 percent increase in calories burned using the interval method is roughly the equivalent of exercising 30 percent longer at the original pace."

To read the full article go to www.NoExcusesWorkouts.com/Book

ARTICLE #3: ASSOCIATED PRESS: INTERVAL TRAINING CAN CUT EXERCISE HOURS SHARPLY

> "People who complain they have no time to exercise may soon need another excuse."
>
> "High-intensity interval training is twice as effective as normal exercise," said Jan Helgerud, an exercise expert at the Norwegian University of Science and Technology. "This is like finding a new pill that works twice as well...We should immediately throw out the old way of exercising."

To read the full article go to www.NoExcusesWorkouts.com/Book

WHY YOU SHOULD NOT DO INTERVALS EVERY DAY

You now realize how powerful Interval Workouts are for cranking up your metabolism, maximizing your calorie burning, strengthening your lungs and heart, and improving your health. So naturally I'm guessing you're wondering why I only suggest that you do them every other day.

The reason you should only be doing three intervals per week is because your heart is a muscle, and it needs recovery time to get stronger. So only do Intervals every other day with days of limiting how high you get your heart rate (while doing the No Excuses Workouts) in between.

Let me explain with an example: If you did bicep curls every day, all you would do is perpetually exhaust your bicep muscles. When you work a muscle, you aren't getting any stronger during the exercise. The muscle fibers are torn and then they rebuild and get stronger over the next twenty-four to forty-eight hours after the workout. This is when the strength of the muscle increases.

The same principle applies to your heart muscle. You need to give it rest every other day. So your Interval Workouts are your high heart rate days and your do the No Excuses Workouts allow you to keep your heart rate lower for recovery purposes. For this reason you should alternate your No Excuses Workouts with your Interval Training.

I know we all think that if a little bit of something is helpful that more must be better. But in this case, it isn't true.

THE POWER OF USING A HEART RATE MONITOR

Do you currently use a Heart Rate Monitor while exercising? If so, than you know how amazing a tool this "coach on your wrist" can be. If you're not currently using this tool, I want you to seriously consider investing in one.

Exercising without a Heart Rate Monitor is like driving from Boston to LA without a map. Yes, you may get there, but you'll surely waste a lot of time along the way.

Don't be intimidated - today's Heart Rate Monitors are easy to set up, and most start with the tap of a few buttons. Yes, it's that easy.

Using a Heart Rate Monitor replaces guesses about your effort level with facts. It guides you in making sure you're working out hard enough and guards you from pushing yourself too hard, risking injury and burnout in the process.

Using a Heart Rate Monitor is like having a coach on your wrist, telling you to speed up or slow down. As you watch your heart rate numbers improve your motivation to continue striving goes up significantly.

Here is the order of least to most effective ways to maximize your fitness and weight-loss results:

1) Do any movement.
2) Do intervals using perceived exertion.
3) Do intervals using a heart-rate monitor.
4) Do personalized intervals using a Heart Rate Monitor.

Consider investing in a Heart Rate Monitor today. As you now know, a Heart Rate Monitor will multiply the effectiveness of your routine. I want you to win by maximizing every minute of every workout you do! Take it from me, using a Heart Rate Monitor is the way to go.

WHY STRENGTH TRAINING IS SO IMPORTANT

Most people blow off strength training because they think it's boring or that they don't burn enough calories. But as you're about to learn, you can make these workouts fun while also cranking up your metabolism!

Here are some of the benefits you can expect from your Strength Training Program. You will:

- Fight off osteoporosis
- Avoid injuries (especially back pain)
- Improve your posture
- Burn more fat at rest
- Tone your body

HOW TO MAKE YOUR NO EXCUSES WORKOUTS FUN

Here is my suggestion for how you can make your No Excuses Workouts fun:

- After every one or two exercises, do thirty to sixty seconds of fun movement to get your heart rate up and turn the workout into a Mini-Interval Workout. Dance, walk in place, run in place, do jumping jacks, pretend you are a skier or boxer - do anything that gets your heart rate up between exercises.

Please note that you shouldn't be hammering too hard because your heart muscle needs rest after the previous day's Interval Workout.

By incorporating these 30-60 second cardio moves into your Strength Training Routine, you'll burn more calories, sweat more, and most likely have a lot more fun!

THE IMPORTANCE OF A STRONG CORE

Having a strong core is important for many reasons beyond looking good. It helps you:

- Avoid injury
- Protect your back
- Maintain good posture
- Perform better in everyday activities and sports

Most people think of a strong core as only having strong abs, but that isn't the case. In order to build a strong core, you need to engage and work your lower back as well. That's why the No Excuses Workouts include back extensions. We want to make sure that your entire core—abs, obloquies, and lower back are all strong.

By consistently doing the No Excuses workout, you'll build a strong core that will help you be more safe and pain-free while making you proud of your toned midsection.

THE 5-MINUTE RULE

Ninety percent of the battle with doing a workout is just getting started. This one simple tip may be the most important thing you learn in this book, so don't let this opportunity pas you by.

Here is how the 5-Minute Rule Solves this common challenge:

You agree to exercise for five minutes no matter what. On the days you're not feeling it and want to blow off your workout, please just commit to moving for five minutes. Most of the time once you start the workout you begin to feel better, and all of a sudden five minutes leads to ten minutes leads to you doing your full workout. And that can be a powerful personal-growth opportunity because you feel great about yourself for fighting through your resistance and coming out the other side.

Follow the 5-Minute Rule and it will be a game-changer for you. Trust me, it works!

CHAPTER 15: HEALTHY EATING IS SIMPLE (NOT EASY)

POSITIVE WEIGHT LOSS, NOT DIETING

As we discussed at the beginning of the book, diets don't work! Not because you are some weirdo who lacks willpower. It is because if we try to make drastic changes to our eating or exercise habits we inevitably bend back. So instead of being fooled into thinking a diet will work focus on what you *can* do to lose weight and keep it off:

- Watch your portions (including not having seconds).
- Never skip meals (especially breakfast).
- Only have dessert once per week (yes, I'm serious).
- Limit drinks other than water to one per day (e.g., soda, beer, wine).
- Eat healthy snacks midmorning and midafternoon.
- Stay hydrated.

- Crank up your metabolism by exercising consistently—especially doing Interval Workouts.

The weight-loss equation is clear: to effectively lose weight and keep it off, you need to burn more calories than you consume. To lose one pound, you need to burn 3,500 more calories than you consume. To lose one pound per week (or fifty-two pounds in a year), you need to burn 500 more calories than you consume each day. If you base your nutritional choices on this equation, you are well on your way to healthy weight loss.

ARE YOUR PORTIONS ROBBING YOU OF RESULTS?

The truth is that we all eat too much. We probably only need about three-quarters of a plate of food, but most people eat a full plate and then go back for seconds. In addition, the portion sizes at restaurants are making it even more challenging. Unfortunately, since we have all gotten used to eating large portions at restaurants we seem to have taken that unhealthy habit home.

Instead of eating everything on your plate, eat until you are no longer hungry. This will make a huge difference when it comes to losing weight and keeping it off.

Let me share a few frightening facts about Americans and their portion sizes (these figures are from research from Tufts University):

- Americans consume more calories per person than any country in the world.
- In 1970 the average American ate 2,170 calories per day.
- In 2000 the average American ate 2,700 calories per day. That is a 530-calorie increase (a 25 percent rise in calorie consumption) in thirty years.
- In 2008, the average American ate 3,330 calories per day. That is a 1,160-calorie increase (a 53 percent rise in calorie consumption) in thirty-eight years.

Is it any wonder that America is in the midst of an Obesity Epedemic?

To get you started on reigning in your portions, I want you to start eating three-quarters of what you normally eat during breakfast, lunch, and dinner. Yes, I'm serious. It may help to write down everything you eat for a week (this is usually shocking). As with all changes, this will take some time to get used to, but eventually it'll start to feel "normal."

As always when you start to make changes with your health, please don't take an all-or-nothing approach! Just keep it simple and take action. Take control of your portions today, and you'll be amazed what this does for your weight loss, energy, and health.

WHY SKIPPING MEALS IS COUNTERPRODUCTIVE

Many people try to skip meals to lose weight. Although it seems like it should work, it's actually counterproductive. Skipping meals or not taking in enough calories leaves you with low energy, compromises your health, and definitely doesn't help with losing weight.

When your body is deprived of needed nutrients, its response is to store food until future meals. This response dates back to the early days of existence when food was scarce and people often needed to survive without a lot of food. The body starts anticipating this cycle and stores food in order to avoid starvation in the future. So although you take in fewer calories, you actually store more calories, and you also slow down your metabolism. These negative health, energy, and metabolism-slowing effects cancel out the reduction in calories.

So what should you do?

The best way to keep your metabolism elevated (not to mention help you maintain energy throughout the day and keep your immune system strong) is to eat every two to three hours. Ideally you'll have three full meals—breakfast, lunch, and dinner—and then have healthy snacks of one hundred to three hundred calories in between meals. This approach will actually help you lose more weight, even through you may find it counter-intuitive.

If you're one of the seventy million Americans currently on a diet, I propose that you try this new approach: eat every two to three hours, watch your portions, take in plenty of water, and crank up your metabolism by doing Interval Workouts. This system will enable you to drop the word "diet" and help you adopt a healthy and sustainable new lifestyle. You and your health are worth it.

DESSERT: LOSE WEIGHT BY HAVING IT ONCE PER WEEK

I want you to start limiting yourself to one dessert per week—no excuses! This will be tough at first, but you'll get used it after just a few weeks.

You should pick one day during the week to be your special dessert night. That way, you'll cut back on a lot of unhealthy calories and enjoy the dessert that much more. If you have dessert every night, it's not that exciting. But if you only have it once per week, it's a real treat!

If cutting back to one dessert per week seems impossible, start by having dessert one less day per week. Then, each week deduct another dessert day until you make it down to one dessert per week.

I suggest on your non-dessert nights that you have a healthy yogurt. This keeps you from being hungry in the evening and lying in bed reading with your stomach growling.

Here's an example of how much this can help you lose or maintain weight. If you're currently having dessert seven nights per week, you're probably taking in around 3,500 calories in desserts per week. When (notice I'm saying "when" and not "if") you cut back to one night of dessert per week plus healthy yogurts on the other nights, you will be cutting approximately 2,400 calories from your weekly intake!

Remember, to lose one pound, you have to have a 3,500-calorie difference between calories burned and calories consumed. So cutting 2,400 calories from your weekly total should lead to 36 pounds lost in one year!

LIMIT YOUR SODA INTAKE

How many sodas are you drinking per day? Please be honest with yourself! Starting today, I want you to decrease your soda intake to one soda per day! Yes, I'm serious. As explained by an article titled "Soda Making Americans Drink Themselves Fat," sodas are a huge contributor to Americans' continued battle with obesity. Here are a few alarming quotes from the article:

- "Liquid candy' to detractors, sweetened soft drinks are so ubiquitous that they contribute about 10 percent of the calories in the American diet, according to government data."
- "Highly concentrated starches and sugars promote overeating, and the granddaddy of them all is sugar-sweetened beverages," said Dr. David Ludwig, a Harvard endocrinologist who runs the Optimal Weight for Life Program at Children's Hospital in Boston. The sugar in soda pop not only provides a massive dose of calories but also triggers a vicious appetite cycle, said Ludwig, who wrote *Ending the Food Fight* about healthy eating for children.

The article does a much better job than I can of explaining the details, so please give it a read by going to www.NoExcusesWorkouts.com/Book

Changing old habits can be tough, so take it one step at a time. Remember, I'm not telling you can't have soda anymore—just to limit yourself to one per day. Try to replace this habit with water. If you're worried about staying awake, then focus on nailing your Interval Workouts and No Excuses Workouts throughout the week. I can guarantee you that your energy levels will increase, and exercise is a more sustainable and natural way of staying energized throughout the day.

HOW LIMITING ALCOHOL CAN HELP YOU LOSE 30 POUNDS IN 1 YEAR

Now that I have officially lost the popularity contest by asking you to decrease your desserts and sodas, I figure I might as well go for a third important and unpopular topic: alcohol consumption.

Don't let wine or beer ruin your progress. I want you to try to limit yourself to one glass of wine or one beer per night so that you don't cancel out all the hard work you're doing.

Please look at the following comparison that shows how much limiting your wine consumption can positively affect your weight-loss efforts:

- One six-ounce glass of wine is around 150 calories.
- Drinking one glass per day = 1,050 calories per week or 54,600 calories per year.
- Drinking two glasses per day = 2,100 calories per week or 109,200 calories per year.
- Drinking three glasses per day = 3,150 calories per week or 163,800 calories per year.

And since you need to burn 3,500 more calories than you consume to lose one pound, decreasing your wine intake from two or three glasses to one glass per day can have a substantial impact on your weight-loss results!

- If you cut back from two glasses to one, you could lose 15.6 pounds in one year!
- If you cut back from three glasses to one, you could lose 31.2 pounds in one year!

Let me give a real life example of this powerful principle in action: I once had a personal-training client who was crushing her Interval Workouts, doing great strength training, and practicing solid nutrition. But she wasn't losing weight. Eventually she admitted she was drinking three glasses of wine per night. After making the decision to limit herself to one glass per night, she proceeded to lose twenty-two pounds and now looks and feels like a rock star.

Do you drink more than one glass of wine or more than one beer per night? Limit yourself to one glass of wine or beer per night so that you can maximize your fitness and weight-loss results. You and your health are worth it!

EAT HEALTHY SNACKS

Snacking is important! Remember, by eating every two to three hours, you keep your metabolism elevated and cranking along. Think of it like placing logs on a fire every couple of hours to keep it burning. Here are some quick and easy snack ideas:

- banana
- apple or celery with some peanut butter (preferably organic)
- carrots
- granola bar
- peanut-butter crackers (the ones with no trans fats)

- a Clif Bar, Balance Bar, or other all-natural energy bar
- a bowl of healthy cereal
- a small handful of unsalted nuts
- pretzels

I suggest you add your list of healthy snacks to your grocery list and set yourself up for healthy snacking by stocking your cabinets. Buying in bulk will save you money and help you avoid running out of healthy snacks at the same time.

STAY HYDRATED: HOW MUCH WATER DO YOU REALLY NEED?

Our bodies are mostly water, so it's imperative for your health and for your workouts that you stay hydrated. Plus, staying hydrated helps you feel fuller and can therefore help you maintain healthy portions.

I have used the following approach to guide people on proper hydration for over a decade and they have had great results:

The general rule is to drink approximately sixty-four ounces of water per day. I suggest taking in an additional ounce per minute of exercise. So if you do a thirty-minute workout, you should take in approximate ninety-four ounces of water. Since consuming sixty-four ounces is a general estimate I suggest you drink enough water throughout the day so that you're going to the bathroom at least once every one to two hours. As long as that's happening and your urine isn't bright yellow then you should be all set.

Use water as part of your overall "get healthy" plan, as the benefits are very important!

17 BENEFITS OF DRINKING WATER

1. Composes 75% of your Brain
2. Regulates your body temperature
3. Makes up 83% of your blood
4. Makes up 75% of your muscles
5. Composes 22% of your bones
6. Helps convert food into energy
7. Removes waste and toxins
8. Helps your body absorb nutrients
9. Moistens oxygen for breathing
10. Cushions your joints
11. Helps carry nutrients and oxygen to your cells
12. Improves your productivity at work
13. Natural remedy for headache
14. Relieves fatigue and improves your mood
15. Reduces the risk of cancer

16. Improves your performance during exercise
17. Makes you look younger and healthier

FUEL YOUR BODY FOR SUCCESSFUL WORKOUTS

It's very important that you have something to eat (either a major meal or a healthy snack) within two hours prior to exercising. This will help you maintain your energy throughout your workout and help you avoid that burnout feeling that can come at the end of your workouts.

If you exercise early in the morning, it's important to take in some nutrients (unless you literally start exercising within thirty minutes of waking) prior to working out. Nothing heavy—just something quick like a piece of fruit, a piece of toast, half a bowl of cereal or a granola bar.

It's also important to be well hydrated prior to exercising. Make sure to drink water throughout the one to two hours prior to your workout so that you are hydrated before you start.

Ideally you'll go to the bathroom within the thirty minutes prior to starting your exercise. That is a good sign that you're hydrated—especially if it isn't bright yellow.

It's also important to have a water bottle with you all the time while you exercise, and to get in the habit of taking a sip every five to ten minutes. If you're sweating while exercising (which hopefully you are), then you're losing a lot of water and need to replenish it.

Lastly, it's very important that you eat something (not necessarily a full meal, but at least a healthy snack) within thirty minutes of finishing your workout. This is because your muscles are looking for nutrients to help them start to rebuild and get stronger. The thirty-minute window is the ideal window to give your muscles fuel to start that very important process.

Use the above tips to fuel your body. It will perform better and you will bounce back from workouts faster.

DON'T USE EXERCISE AS AN EXCUSE TO EAT BADLY

You may recall a controversial article that was on the cover of *Time* magazine back in 2010 stating "Why Exercise Won't Make You Thin!" That bold statement was more to sell magazines than to try to argue that exercise doesn't work for weight loss. The core of the article, however, was about how many people use their exercise habits as their excuse to eat badly.

Is that you?

If you've been nailing three Interval Workouts and three No Excuses Workouts each week for at least two weeks and you have not lost weight or lost inches or cranked up your energy, then nutrition is definitely the problem.

If you've been using your exercise as a reason to eat badly or crank up your calorie intake, then I suggest you make a firm and serious commitment to yourself right now to put an end to it.

Here's why: life's too short to spin your wheels.

When you nail your workouts (two steps up the stairs) and then counter that with bad nutrition (two steps back down the stairs), your net fitness and weight loss results are zero.

I want you to take a few minutes right now to honestly ask yourself if you're using exercise as your excuse to eat badly. Being candid with and accountable to yourself will finally allow your rocket to leave the pad!

THE 5 TRIGGERS OF BAD NUTRITIONAL CHOICES

If you look back at the times so far this year that you have made bad nutritional choices, I'm sure that

90 percent of the time the following five things did not happen:

1) You didn't have breakfast within one hour of waking up.
2) You hadn't eaten every two to three hours that day.
3) You weren't well hydrated.
4) You hadn't slept at least seven hours the night before.
5) You hadn't exercised.

Eating badly isn't the product of some weird gene you have; nor is it due to a complete lack of self-control. Most of the time it's simply due to a lack of being aware of the triggers that lead you to making bad choices.

Focus on making these five things happen each day, and you'll not only feel better but your bad nutritional choices will drop considerably. Have fun showing your negative voice that you don't lack willpower and that now you have the tools you need to master your nutrition!

DITCH THE DIET: MY TOP 7 NUTRITION TIPS

Instead of being on some crazy diet that leaves you feeling like you could chew on your arm, follow these seven simple tips and ditch the word "diet" forever:

1) Eat breakfast within one hour of waking up—this kick-starts your metabolism.
2) Drink sixty-four ounces of water per day—you should be going to the bathroom every one to two hours.
3) Eat every two to three hours throughout the day, including healthy snacks midmorning and midafternoon.
4) Limit your portion sizes—no seconds.
5) Limit yourself to one soda per day (ideally zero) and no coffee after noon.
6) Limit yourself to one dessert per week (and have a healthy yogurt on the other six nights).
7) Chew your food until it's liquid—this slows down how quickly you eat and lets you think about how you're fueling your body.

Follow these seven tips, and you'll be pleasantly surprised how much this improves your energy and health.

5 TIPS TO ENJOY HOLIDAY PARTIES

You can have a blast at holiday parties and cookouts without kicking yourself the next morning. Here are my five tips to enjoying holiday parties without overdoing it:

1) Do a solid workout in the morning prior to hosting or going to a party.

2) Eat a healthy snack thirty to sixty minutes prior to the party.
3) Drink plenty of water all day and during the party.
4) Fill at least one-third of your plate with salad or another healthy option.
5) Put your "everything in moderation" hat on.

You can eat fun things in moderation, have fun at the party, and not beat yourself up the next day for hindering your fitness and weight-loss efforts.

6 TIPS FOR HOW TO WIN WHILE EATING OUT

With a little planning and deciding ahead of time that you're going to have a healthy night out, you'll have fun and be proud the next morning. Here are my six tips for how to win while eating out:

1) Look up the restaurant's menu prior to going so that you can look over the healthy options and know what you'll be ordering before you get there.
2) Have a healthy snack ranging from one hundred to three hundred calories within ninety minutes of leaving for the restaurant.
3) Skip participating in the appetizer.
4) Drink plenty of water.

5) Chew your food until it's liquid (this slows down how quickly you eat).
6) If you order dessert, split it with your spouse or friend.

Then smile on the way home from the restaurant as you celebrate how well you did!

PLAY OFFENSE TO WIN THE NUTRITION BATTLE

Most people don't plan for success as far as their nutrition. They wing it, and that rarely works out. Earlier we went over why it's so important to use the Win Tomorrow and Win Today checklists to dial-in healthy habits.

Another great way to play offense and take control of your nutrition is to do the following:

1) Never put together your shopping list on an empty stomach.
2) Never go to a grocery store on an empty stomach.

These two tips may seem overly simple, but 90 percent of the problem with nutrition starts at the grocery store. If you don't put bad foods in your cart, then they aren't available at home for you to make bad choices.

So play offense! Make healthy shopping lists and shop smart, and the likelihood of your buying unhealthy things will drop by ten times. Use this strategy to win!

CHAPTER 16: BE YOUR FAMILY'S CHIEF WELLNESS OFFICER

PUT YOUR OXYGEN MASK ON FIRST

When you fly, the safety presentation always talks about putting your own oxygen mask on prior to helping your kids. This also relates to your health and your kids' health. You need to take care of yourself and be as healthy as possible to be able to do the best job taking care of your kids.

Honestly, think about this for a minute. Skipping breakfast, not having healthy snacks during the morning and afternoon, not staying hydrated, and not working out do not put you in the best spot to be your best!

Parents often put themselves last, even sacrificing their health and wellness because they want to be good parents. They care so much about their kids that they put all their focus and energy into them. However, parents are at their best when they take care of themselves. When a parent is healthy she or he is able to so the best job possible.

Invest some of your valuable time and energy in yourself. Put your oxygen mask on first, and it will pay off many times over for your kids and your whole family.

YOUR TEAM IS FOLLOWING YOUR LEAD

Even when we want to take care of ourselves, staying consistent with workouts and healthy eating is hard work! Our negative voices are constantly hitting us with excuses to blow off our workouts and eat badly. When this happens, I invite you to focus on how much your family (especially your kids) is following your lead.

The only real way to help your kids get healthy is to lead by example. Trying to force exercise or restrictive nutrition on your kids usually backfires.

According to the American Academy of Child and Adolescent Psychiatry:

- A child with one obese parent is 50 percent likely to become an obese adult.

- A child with two obese parents is 80 percent likely to become an obese adult.

As a parent, your weight and lifestyle have a large impact on your child's activity level, eating habits, and outlook on weight. So take the stairs instead of the elevator, park in the farthest spot at the grocery store, and do something active with your kids each day so that you can fit a little exercise into your life. In simple terms, you have to walk the talk as far as living and being healthy.

There are many positive qualities that you work hard to pass on to your children: treating people correctly, a strong work ethic, studying, doing the right thing and so on. But sadly and unfortunately, most Americans also pass on their health and weight problems.

If the idea of having tons of energy and being healthy isn't enough to get you in the game, then get healthy so that your children have a chance to be healthy adults and pass goo health on to your grandchildren.

Remember, our kids become us! If we're active and healthy, they are active and healthy. Unfortunately, the opposite is true. Your negative voice will try to talk you out of the following statement but it is a fact: you are your family's chief wellness officer. Wear that hat proudly and lead your team. Your kids will become healthy and thriving adults if you help them build healthy habits now.

MY HUSBAND IS PROBABLY GOING TO DIE OF A HEART ATTACK

"My husband is probably going to die of a heart attack if he doesn't lose weight." These are the sad words I heard from a women at the gym one day. Her husband weighs three hundred pounds and refuses to make his health a priority. The saddest part is that they have a nine-year-old son who, in the words of his mom, is going to grow up without a father if things don't change.

As I've shared, my dad died of cardiac arrest due to his weight issues, so this is personal and I want to help you out if you're in the same situation as the woman I just mentioned. I gave her a number of suggestions, and I want to share them with you.

Here's a list of ideas of how you can help your spouse lose weight:

1) Limit the amount of unhealthy snacks you buy while food shopping.
2) Buy healthier snacks like granola bars and pretzels to take the place of chips and cookies.
3) Serve smaller portions for dinner, and refuse to serve seconds (in fact, pack the extras up and put them in the fridge after filling each plate).
4) Lead by example by only having dessert once per week and having a yogurt on the other nights.
5) Make your spouse's lunch, which will support healthy eating, control lunch portions and discourage eating out.

6) Lead family walks in the evening and on weekend mornings.

These tips definitely wok, but the #1 way to help your spouse lose weight and get healthy is to lose and get healthy yourself.

GET YOUR FAMILY INVOLVED

Exercising with your kids or spouse is a positive thing to do for many reasons:

- It improves their health (and yours).
- You spend quality time together.
- Exercise can be great for your kids' self-esteem.
- You serve as a healthy role model to your kids.
- You all feel great and proud when you're done.

All that is really required is that you are getting your heart rate up and working your muscles more than sitting down. That's a great and simple way to define exercise for your kids.

Here is a tip, play with your kids. Think about this. Do you play with your kids (throw a ball, play tag or run around) or do you watch them play? Be honest with yourself, this is important.

DINOSAUR HUNTING WITH ALEXANDER AND BENJAMIN

Now I want to give you a great example of an active game that I play with my boys: dinosaur hunting! When Alexander and Benjamin were three and one, I asked them one day if they wanted to hunt for dinosaurs, and they both got huge smiles on their faces.

Here is how we hunt for dinosaurs: we lie on the living room floor with our heads close together, and then I say, "Where do you think the first one is?" Then Alexander names a room in the house, and we crawl on our hands and knees to the spot. He pretends to grab the dinosaur, and we all jump up and run to a chair in our living room. Then Benjamin puts the dinosaur in the chair, and we lie back down on our stomachs with our heads close and figure out where the next one is.

We normally play for five to ten minutes, and it's an absolute blast. And at the same time I get a great workout and the boys are staying active. This is truly a win-win.

Please try dinosaur hunting (or other fun and active games) with your kids. What games can you play with your kids while getting a workout? Tap into the energy of your kids and you will have a blast together!

CHAPTER 17: MOMS, GET BACK TO YOUR PRE-PREGNANCY WEIGHT

DO YOU FEEL GUILTY ABOUT TAKING TIME TO EXERCISE?

Many parents (especially moms) feel guilty about taking time away from their kids to exercise.

But the benefit for your kids of having a parent with tons of energy who is generally in a good mood pays off tenfold. Plus, as we discussed earlier, by being an example of health to your kids, you set them up to be healthy adults who enjoy long lives.

Remember that our kids follow our lead! If we're active and healthy, they're usually active and healthy.

GIVE, GIVE, GIVE

If you're a mom, then you spend every waking moment giving. You're taking care of the kids, the house, the meals, the everything. You are the glue that keeps the house together. Husbands mean well (me included). But we're in right field, and most of us would come apart without our amazing wives.

Spending your entire day giving leaves you with little or no time for yourself. This needs to change! At one point in your life, you and your health were a top priority. Maybe it was in high school or college, or more than likely it was before your first child was born. Moms are the hardest-working people on this earth, and they're also the first ones to remove themselves from their own priority lists.

If you're a mom, you need and deserve to do something uncomfortable: you have to starting giving to yourself without viewing it as depriving your family. You deserve to carve out personal time each day to exercise and invest in your health. Your house won't fall apart and your kids and spouse will end up benefiting from a more energized, healthy, and happy version of you.

You may tell yourself you don't have time and then put your workouts or your health needs off for another day. Soon the days become weeks, then months and then years. I invite you right now to not only put yourself back on your priority list but to move your health and your workouts up to the top (yes, I'm serious). In the near term your kids and spouse may gripe, but in the coming weeks they'll see the positive changes in your energy and mood. Then everyone wins!

So carve out some "me time" each day, and you'll be pleasantly surprised by how much better you feel mentally and physically and how much this benefits your family.

Thanks to all of you moms for keeping our families functioning. You are all rock stars!

TREAT YOURSELF AS WELL AS YOU TREAT YOUR KIDS

If I haven't convinced you to make time for yourself to exercise, consider this: How well do you treat yourself versus how you treat your kids? Would you ever let your kids skip meals, drink limited water throughout the day, avoid physical activity for weeks or months at a time, or not eat anything for five or six hours straight? Honestly, think about this for a minute.

You deserve to treat yourself as well as you treat your kids! Your health is too important not to do this. Consider it as an investment in yourself. Plus, by taking time to invest in your health each day, you'll bring more energy to interact your kids and serve as an example of health and fitness for them to follow.

You and your health are worth it!

WAITING FOR THE IDEAL TIME IS A PIPE DREAM

I know I've mentioned this before, but it's worth repeating here especially for moms. Most people keep telling themselves the same type of stories:

- When things settle down at work, I'll lose the weight.
- When the kids are older, it'll be easier to focus on myself.
- When I invest in a gym membership, I'll start getting fit.
- When things are less stressful, I'll start eating right.

The sad thing is that when we wait for the ideal time to start losing weight and getting fit, it rarely comes.

Our lives are perpetually busy and crazy (especially for moms), and we need to ditch the dream that a magical day in the not-too-far future will happen when everything will line up and we can go for it! If you wait for that day, you'll be waiting forever, and you'll continue to be robbed of becoming who you deserve to be.

In addition to watching my amazing wife be a pillar of strength for our family, I have had the privilege of working with thousands of Moms; Moms who prove day in and day out that they know what it means to be strong when others need them.

Now is your chance to shine your strength in your own direction so that you can re-discover your energy, vitality and health. This program was designed for you, the busy Mom, so let these proven methods be an on-going resource for you to chase down our dreams!

CONCLUSION

Congratulations on working your way through the entire book! I don't need to ask you if you are interested or committed as far as getting fit and losing weight because clearly you are committed!

As I stated at the beginning of the book, the true battleground is in your head and in particular getting your negative voice to zip it. Focus on following my 15 Secrets to Better Health and being in control of your inner-dialogue and you will shock yourself with your results.

NOW is your time and this is your year so hit the gas and go for it!

If you have not already joined the Free No Excuses Team, please go to: http://www.NoExcusesWorkouts.com

If you want more personalized guidance please check out our Online Boot Camps (where you can workout live with me and our other coaches right in your living room) by going to the above website. For $20 off one Boot Camp, use Coupon Code Kona10140619.

Thanks for giving me this opportunity to guide you to being your best!